CONTENTS

RESTRUCTURING THE HEALTH SERVICE

TOM HELLER

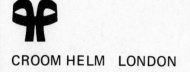

CROOM HELM   LONDON

© 1978 William Temple Foundation

Croom Helm Ltd, 2-10 St John's Road, London SW11

British Library Cataloguing in Publication Data

Heller, Tom
  Restructuring the health service.
  1. Health services administration – Great
  Britain
  2. Great Britain – National Health Service
  I. Title
  362.1'0941   RA395.G6

ISBN 0-85664-583-4

Printed and bound in Great Britain by
REDWOOD BURN LIMITED
Trowbridge & Esher

FOREWORD

The William Temple Foundation is an independent unit for consultation and research concerned with the relation between Christian faith, the churches and the social order. In order to gain an understanding which could lead to response in this area it has been necessary to study selected important institutions or critical disturbance areas. The object of the study is to develop an account of what is involved in a particular institution or problem area to the point where what is going on in the institution and what is happening to human beings as a result can be perceived and elucidated. The hypothesis is that this will provide a basis for developing insights into possible Christian responses in our current institutional crises and social disturbances.

The areas in which the Foundation is attempting to develop this approach at present include the operations of a heavy production industry, the problems of underprivileged young people and the labour market, the issues arising in community development and the effects of current economic limitations on the health service. This book is a report arising from our studies in this last area.

The hypothesis on which the Foundation's National Health Service project was launched was that the decisive discovery of strict limits on the resources which could be made available for the NHS provided an urgent opportunity for re-assessing what we ought to mean by 'health', what sort of service should therefore be developed in and by society and how this service should be related to the community, the health of whose members it was supposed to serve. Funds were obtained to employ Dr Tom Heller for an initial period of two years and the University of East Anglia agreed to his continuing as Visiting Senior Research Associate based in their School of Development Studies. The material which he has prepared was first consolidated into a submission to the Royal Commission on the National Health Service and has now been slightly revised and expanded to form the present publication.

As far as the aims of the William Temple Foundation are concerned, the work represents stage one only in a particular project. It does not contain and it is not intended to contain any reflections or suggestions about the relation of Christian faith to the institutional, political and human problems outlined. It is presented as an analytical and reflective contribution in its own right to our present concerns about society and about health care provision.

Attempts are being made to carry on the project in two directions. On the one hand, ways and means are being sought to relate the diagnosis developed in this book to a practical experiment to develop appropriate responses on the ground. We aim at developing some experimental work for enabling a community to play a bigger part in its own health care and so to assist in the evolution of some alternative models for health care and some consequent modifications in the services providing health care. On the other hand the Foundation is working at developing the implications and applications both for Christian faith and arising from Christian faith with regard to the working of institutions and their effects on human beings, as exposed by the work which has been done so far. What is aimed at is a continuing interplay between experimentation and reflection which will maintain what it is hoped will be a creative and revealing tension. On the one hand the experimentation must be able to continue without the participants being required to identify with a particular faith-stance. On the other hand it must not be possible to escape the facing of the more fundamental questions of what human beings are actually about while attempting to deal with particular needs or combat particular obstacles and distortions.

David E. Jenkins
Director
William Temple Foundation
Manchester

PREFACE

There can be no doubt that this is a time of rapid change for the
National Health Service. Many of its services appear to be under
considerable strain and there is evidence of tension between the
various sectional interests involved in the health service. The William
Temple Foundation has produced this study of the NHS
precisely because it has no partisan involvement with any of the
groups directly involved in producing the service. However, the group
has attempted throughout to present a new analysis of the basic
dynamics of the health service as seen by the total community of
potential and actual consumers/clients/patients.

1 DECISION-MAKING IN THE HEALTH SERVICE

One of the basic problems facing the National Health Service is the relationships of power within it. The various sectional interests can present their views, but who represents the patient or potential consumer, and what really is in the best interest of the community as a whole? Thus there is a need for an independent study of the NHS. This book is critical of the two major decision-making groups within the health service, the administration/management and the medical profession. The criticism is intended to be constructive rather than destructive, and it is intended to lead to a movement towards much closer co-operation between these two groups and to a very real involvement of the community in the development of a healthy society.

It should be made clear that these criticisms of the major decision-making groups within the NHS are levelled at the system of decision-making, rather than at the individuals within that system. Throughout the course of the study the author has come into contact with large numbers of doctors and administrators, many of whom, as individuals, have been concerned with much the same issues as are explored here. However, it is central to this analysis that the individuals within the system are constrained such that the potential for individual action is severely limited.

The shape of the National Health Service has been determined by the conflict between the two major decision-making groups within it, the medical profession and the management/administration. The interests of these two groups are really quite different. The medical profession wants to keep in control and resents and resists attempts to introduce the rational management of its affairs that would be required by the managers to create an 'efficient' system. This dynamic has created enormous distortions in the Service which are described in Chapter 4 and also prevents these distortions from being overcome. More importantly, this basic power dynamic within the NHS has meant that the protagonists have lost sight of the people for whom it is intended. Individuals as patients and communities of potential patients have little effective voice to determine the sort of health service that they need. Similarly, the bulk of the ordinary workers within the NHS (now the largest single employer in the country employing over 900,000 people) are without any meaningful power when it comes to decision-making to determine the structure and functioning of the Service.

The Power of the Administration

The power of administration is analysed in Chapter 2. This power can be shown by observing the manner in which it 'consults' the people, both at national and at local level. At national level the Department of Health and Social Security has published (1976) a consultative document called *Priorities for Health and Personal Social Services.* Although this document describes itself as a 'new departure', detailed analysis of its contents shows that no new priorities are actually projected and that both the contents of the document and the procedure used for consultation are being used as a facade *instead of* real consultation.[1] Similarly, at local levels the administration often treats individuals, local interest groups, and the new Community Health Councils in an offhand manner that emphasises the lack of influence these groups have over the affairs of the NHS.

The power of administrators as a group can also be shown by the recent growth in the numbers of administrators employed in the NHS. In the ten years before the reorganisation of the NHS in 1974, the numbers employed increased by 65 per cent, while the number of doctors increased by 21 per cent, and domestics, etc., by only 2 per cent.[2] During the process of reorganisation the power of this group was once again demonstrated by its ability to increase its numbers and its control over the organisation of the Service.[3]

The management and administration of the health service seem to suffer from a very limited concept of health and to rely on an exclusively administrative approach to the nation's health. The 'problems' of the nation's health are perceived as being largely amenable to the ministrations of the statutory services if only they can be 'delivered' efficiently enough. This approach presumes that there will be a satisfactory outcome for the nation's health if, and when, the various norms and guidelines are met. The Department of Health is constrained by this very limited model and its concerns appear to be with producing some sort of equity between geographic regions, bringing services up to some arbitrary guidelines and a general striving for cost-effectiveness and efficiency. None of these aims are to be decried as such, but all of them put together can only contribute marginally to the health of the nation, however defined. In addition, all these aims rely on a dominant management which is able to achieve these aims and which must outweigh the immediate interests of NHS employees, including members of the caring professions, and which also relegates individual and community-based decisions to a position of comparatively minor importance.

This limited concept of health, in fact, ignores the evidence concerning the relationship between health services and the measurable levels of health within the community. Various historical and international studies have shown that the organisation of, and expenditure on, health services bears little or no relation to the levels of health found in a community.[4] Furthermore, the *caring* functions of the statutory services have been shown to be of comparatively minor importance compared with the volume of caring that is done in the community by families, friends and various informal and voluntary networks.[5] All this is not to suggest that there should be no statutory health services, but that the current ideology of the administration appears to avoid putting these services into correct perspective. In practice, this would mean that the *caring* functions of the statutory services would have to be reorientated to provide support for the informal systems of caring for people in the community, while the *curative* functions would be restricted largely to interventions of proven effectiveness, and both would be distributed according to need.

The Power of the Medical Profession

The medical profession wields enormous power and resists any attempts to erode its autonomy. However, in pursuing its own ends, the profession is not necessarily acting in the best interests of the health service or of the community as a whole; this is detailed in Chapter 3. Insistence on total autonomy has given rise to the current situation, in which the treatment for similar conditions differs widely and apparently depends only on the whims of the doctor in charge. The variation in days spent in hospital for the treatment of similar conditions is the simplest example where savings could be made by the use of a medical audit or some guidelines for doctors on patients' management.[6]

There are no really effective sanctions against members of the medical profession, and the complaints procedure for both hospitals and the general practitioner services are heavily weighted in favour of the doctors.[7] The doctors themselves sit in judgement over their own colleagues and, even in cases of gross negligence which are dealt with by the General Medical Council, the panel consists largely of other doctors.

The medical profession remains largely orientated towards the technological components of medical practice. Medical education focuses on the advanced technological specialties, and medical students therefore aspire to join these specialties, which naturally attract the greatest kudos and the bulk of the resources of the health service.

In addition, the profession is very aggressive over protecting its own financial interests. This can be seen in the fight to retain private facilities in the National Health Service, although the maintenance of these pay beds costs the NHS more money than it receives in revenue from them, and this practice is to the detriment of the majority of the population, who cannot afford private treatment. The increasingly aggressive wage bargaining stance and frequent threats of strike action detract from the amount of money that is available for actually providing services for patients. An example of this can be taken from within the East Anglian region which has always been very poorly provided with resources. In 1976/7 the region was awarded additional 'development funds' to bring the services up to the standards of the other regions. However, a large portion of these funds (over 50 per cent of the funds available for the Cambridgeshire area, for instance) has gone to pay the increased salaries of the junior hospital doctors.

In no sense are the decisions of the profession made in partnership with the administration, or, more particularly, with any decision-making apparatus within the community. This does not mean that the decisions taken by the profession are never in the interest of the community, but that they are taken on a unilateral basis.

It is not suggested that the medical profession should surrender all its power, status and autonomy, but simply that it should consider a new sort of relationship with the community it purports to serve, whereby decision-making is a matter of co-operation rather than unilateral action. This relationship should naturally extend to the level of individual doctors dealing with individual members of the community. It does appear highly illogical for the medical profession to attempt to keep to itself knowledge about disease processes, etc., at the same time as it bemoans the fact that so many consultations are for apparently trivial reasons. The task of the medical profession in the future should certainly include the specialised treatment of those who have become ill, but should increasingly be orientated to teaching the community how to stay healthy and how to cope with simple ailments as they arise. Some of the problems of re-orienting medical perspectives are discussed in Chapter 6.

Distortions in the Health Service

The power dynamic between the two groups described above, in addition to the historical inheritance of services dating from the start

of the NHS, has led to the development of the severe distortions
detailed in the description of the system in Chapter 4. This shows that

(1) In many geographical areas there is a real deficiency in the
standards and availability of quite ordinary services of all types.

(2) People suffering from some sorts of illness (mainly chronic and
psychiatric illnesses and the effects of old age) receive a standard of
service that is much lower than desirable, and much lower than that
generally offered to those suffering from acute illness.[8]

(3) The caring services as a whole are fragmented such that it is
difficult for those in need of such services to understand or to apply
for the range of services that might be of benefit to them.[9]

(4) Those most in need of services are the least likely to have them
easily available. In particular, a class analysis of the services shows that
the members of social classes iv and v have access to services that are of
generally lower standard, although the members of these social classes
certainly suffer from an increased burden of mortality and morbidity.[10]

(5) The health and caring services as presently organised have only a
minor role in caring for people when they are actually in need.[11]

(6) Decisions on the service are taken far away from those who are
affected by these decisions. This applies to individuals when they are
sick and also to whole communities when considerations of service
development are made. Similarly, those working in the NHS often find
themselves remote from decision-making.

(7) Preventive services are underfinanced, under-researched and
underdeveloped compared with the services concerned with the
treatment of acute illness that might have been prevented in the first
place.

(8) Chapter 7 shows that the shape of the health service described
here has become the accepted norm for the majority of the rest of the
world, and that in the developing countries the effects of the adoption
of tnis type of service are particularly devastating.

(9) Wherever in the world health services of this shape have been
introduced, there is no good evidence that they are effective in reducing
the levels of disease in that country.[12]

Creating a Community-Orientated Health Service

The final chapter concludes that none of these distortions can be
eliminated until the relationships of power within the NHS are altered
such that the consumers/community have a real voice in the service that
is provided, and any movement in that direction must be supported.

This will involve the development of Community Health Councils with the ability to ensure that the real needs of their community are actually met. In addition, the services themselves should become orientated to serve the consumers, for example there should be patients' committees with both power and responsibility as part of each group practice of general practitioners. In addition, pilot projects should be developed to explore different relationships between professionals and the community and new methods of communication between the various branches of the caring services.

There is, in addition, a myriad of more detailed reforms that could be suggested for the improvement of the health service. These would include an improved system of redistribution of resources between geographical regions, types of disease and social classes. Also there are many improvements that could be made to the training programmes of the professional groups, such that the sort of concerns detailed in this short study would receive attention during the student period. Much needs to be done with regard to the development of methods of control over professional power, spending power and complaints procedures as well as the development of administrative machinery that is more democratic, more accountable and more open. However, is is unlikely that any of these will actually be implemented in such a way as to bring about a real change in the service until there is a shift in the relationships of power away from the professionals and the professional managers and towards the people for whom the service is intended.

Notes and References

1. Department of Health and Social Services (DHSS), *Priorities for Health and Personal Social Services* (HMSO, London, 1976). For a very detailed criticism of the consultative document, see the pamphlet *Whose Priorities?*, Radical Statistics Health Group, c/o BSSRS, 9 Poland Street, London W1 (price 45p + 15p).
2. House of Commons written answer, 29 October 1975.
3. Institute of Health Service Studies, *New Bottles, Old Wine?* (Hull University, 1975).
4. B. Abel-Smith, *Value for Money in Health Services* (Heinemann, London, 1976).
5. M. Bayley, *Mental Handicap and Community Care* (Routledge and Kegan Paul, London, 1973).
6. A.L. Cochrane, *Effectiveness and Efficiency* (Nuffield Provincial Hospitals Trust, London, 1971).
7. M. Stacey, 'Consumer Complaints in the British NHS', *Social Science and Medicine*, vol.8 (1974), p.429.
8. P. Townsend, 'Inequality and the Health Service', *Lancet* (1971), vol.1, p.405.

9. *Going Home?* Report of the Continuing Care Project (Age Concern, Liverpool, 1975).

10. J.T. Hart, 'The Inverse Care Law', *Lancet* (1971), vol.1, p.405.

11. P. Pasker, 'Inter-relationship of Different Sectors of the Total Health and Social Services System', *Community Medicine* (1971), vol.126, pp.272-6X.

12. T.D. Heller, 'Some Dynamics and Dilemmas of Medical Care', Internationale Entwicklung, Austrian Foundation for Development Research 1976 /IV. p.13. Reprint available from School of Development Studies, University of East Anglia, Norwich NR4 7TJ.

2 THE ADMINISTRATION OF THE HEALTH SERVICE

There is no doubt that the administration and management of the
health service is becoming increasingly complex and costly.
Administration in the East Anglian Region alone (the lowest spending
region on administration) came to over £9.6 million in 1975/6, which
is equivalent to approximately 14 per cent of the total health services
budget for the region (see Table 2.1). In addition, central administration
costs an additional 0.6 per cent of the total health and personal social
services budget.[1]

The number of administrators has risen faster than the number of
employees in any other sector within the health service (see Table 2.2).

During the reorganisation of the health service in 1974,
administrative costs grew particularly rapidly, as was shown in a survey
in the Humberside region (see Table 2.3). It was estimated that in that
region £173,000 of the total £250,000 costs of reorganisation went on
additional salaries for employees in the administrative and finance
departments.

These statistics demonstrate the power of administrators as a group
to increase their importance relative to the other groups within the
service. However, the statistics cannot demonstrate whether current
spending on administration is too high, too low or just about right, or
give any evidence regarding the quality or effectiveness of the
administration of the service.

One indication of the effectiveness of the administration is how well
the general policy statements of the administration are translated into
action. For example, various general policy statements have been issued
by the administration indicating that increasing priority will be given
to preventive services and services for the mentally handicapped and
mentally ill (see Tables 2.4, 2.5 and 2.6). These priorities have been the
explicit policy of the administration virtually since the inception of
the National Health Service, and yet they have never been translated
into an increased proportion of the budget spent on these particular
services. For example, in 1971 the major statement of government
policy promised 'That particular emphasis will be placed on reducing
the inequalities between regions and on improvement of conditions in
hospitals and services provided for patients such as the mentally

18

Table 2.1.   Administrative Costs, East Anglian Region: 1975/6

	£
Regional tier	2,632,541
Area and district tiers	3,534,400
Family practitioner administration	421,041
Community health councils	62,390
School and community services	211,015
Hospital administration	2,777,792
	9,639,179

Source: East Anglia Regional Health Authority, 'Revenue Allocations 1975/6'.

Table 2.2.   Growth of Number of Employees with the National
             Health Service 1964-1974

	1964	1974	% increase
Doctors and consultants	52,085	63,110	+ 21%
Nurses	212,366	289,956	+ 37%
Domestics, etc.	171,214	175,217	+ 2%
Administration and clerical	48,016	79,114	+ 65%

Source: House of Commons Written Answers, 29 October 1975.

Table 2.3.   Cost of Reorganisation: Humberside Region

	Number		%	£ cost
Grade	before	after	difference	per year
Senior admin.	36	48	+ 33%	66,000
Junior and middle admin.	82	100	+ 22%	54,000
Finance staff	39	54	+ 39%	53,500
Nursing officers (and above)	206	218	+ 6%	25,000
Community medicine specialists	10	9	−10%	no change
Other costs				51,500
				£250,000

Source: Institute of Health Service Studies, *New Bottle, Old Wine?* (Hull
    University, 1975).

Table 2.4. Spending on Preventive Services

	£m	Spending as % of NHS total
1973/4 outturn	15	0.41
1975/6 provisional	15	0.38
1979/80 projection	17	0.39

Source: DHSS, *Priorities for Health and Personal Social Services* (HMSO, London, 1976).

Table 2.5. NHS Capital Expenditure on Services for the Mentally Handicapped

	1970/1	1971/2	1972/3	1973/4	1974/5
Total £000s	119,118	151,466	183,066	204,425	237,000
Services for the mentally handicapped £000s	6,450	7,503	8,517	8,584	8,741
% to services for the mentally handicapped	5.40%	4.95%	4.65%	4.19%	3.70%

Source: House of Commons Parliamentary Questions 21 and 22 May 1975.

Table 2.6. Revenue Expenditure on Services for the Mentally Ill

	1964/5	1967/8	1970/1	1973/4
Total £000s	526,138	667,350	940,616	1,461,574
Services for the mentally ill £000s	67,870	79,841	106,332	164,699
% to services for the mentally ill	12.90%	11.97%	11.30%	11.26%

Source: House of Commons Parliamentary Questions 21 and 22 May 1975.

handicapped and mentally ill, the elderly and younger chronic sick.'[2]

This apparent inability to translate policy into practice might be due to ineffectiveness whereby the administration is attempting to carry out its policies, but is thwarted by various political constraints. This has been documented for the reallocation of resources within one region,[3] and a similar fate can be predicted for the general priorities now being advocated by the DHSS. Detailed consideration of *Priorities for Health and Personal Social Services,* Consultative Document, published in 1976 by the DHSS, shows that, although the DHSS put forward a plausible and logical scheme for the reallocation of resources between the various sectors of the service, in practice they have not got full control over this reallocation.[4] The readjustment of priorities is dependent on considerations of control over manpower, the medical profession, local authorities and the internal machinery of the NHS administration. Any attempted readjustment will certainly be resisted by various powerful factions within the NHS and outside it.

These considerations must surely be well known to the NHS administration, yet their policy document does not fully discuss any of these implications, and they present their priorities as if they can be implemented using the present structure and controls over the system.

Manpower Considerations

The consultative document states that over 70 per cent of the current expenditure for health and personal social services is on staff salaries and wages.[5] This proportion has risen rapidly following the Halsbury Committee report[6] on pay for nurses which added over £170 million to the NHS wages bill, while the fifth review body proposals for doctors' and dentists' pay (1975) added a further £134 million per annum.[7] The wages bill for ancillary workers of all types has also been rapidly expanded recently. Wages and salaries in the hospital and community health services rose by 43 per cent between November 1973 and November 1974, and this has been the major reason for the percentage of GNP devoted to the NHS rising from 4.9 per cent in 1973 to 5.4 per cent in 1975.[8]

Without arguing the merits or demerits of these salary increases, the figures suggest strongly that the positive or negative growth of the various sectors within the health and personal social services is also very largely determined by the labour force structure and the level of wage settlements within the various sectors. It is therefore vital for any policy document which attempts to determine relative priorities between the various sectors to enter fully into the manpower implications inherent in the realignment of resources.

For example, without large elements of manpower redeployment the sectors of the services with the greatest proportion of workers receiving the largest increments in pay will grow faster than other sectors, whatever the stated government priorities. Unfortunately, these vital considerations are only briefly mentioned in the consultative document: 'It will also be necessary for some staff to be redeployed, with their agreement, so that the new priorities can be achieved.'[9] There is, as yet, no positive evidence that staff will agree to deployment. In particular, medical staff in the past have shown a marked reluctance to practise in exactly those sectors that have been selected for priority in this document. Consultant posts in psychiatric, geriatric, and community medicine remain unfilled.

The unions representing ancillary personnel have yet to be approached with the details of the exact implications of these adjustments in priorities for their staffs.

Problems of Medical Autonomy

The medical profession commands the majority of spending power within the health service and has always tended to resist any attempts by the administration to control or rationalise its spending. The variations between doctors treating the same condition have been amply demonstrated and are a major difficulty with regard to planning and budgeting. For example, the average length of hospital stay for surgery in the Liverpool region for varicose veins varied from 2 to 10 days, for haemorrhoids from 2 to 12 days and for hernia from 1 to 12 days.[10] Similar evidence is recorded in the literature on the prescription of medicine, the use of X rays and pathological investigations.[11]

The British Medical Association rejects any form of control over these variations by the administrators of the NHS,[12] and the Merrison Committee report on the regulation of the medical profession stated:

> It [the medical profession] must be independent of the providers of the Country's health service, and it ought not to be the creature of Government. . .We take the view that the medical profession should be largely self-regulated.[13]

Without entering this debate in any further detail, it would, however, seem unlikely that fine adjustment of priorities between the various sectors of the service will be possible in the future without some measure of control of the spending power of individual doctors. The consultative document only states:

> Decisions on clinical practice concerning individual patients are and must continue to be the responsibility of the clinician concerned. But it is hoped that this document will encourage further scrutiny by the professions of the resources used by different treatment regimes.[14]

In the realms of primary care this inability to control the spending power of the medical profession turns the planning exercise into a simple forecast of what the expenditure will be. 'In general it is not proposed to intervene in the natural development of the primary care services, as determined by demand and professional response to it.'[15]

Because of the almost total lack of control in this sector, expenditure is forecast to rise quicker than in the general and acute hospital sector, 3.7 per cent as opposed to 1.2 per cent per annum. This decision is rationalised in the statement that 'this increase should make possible some reduction in referral to the hospital services.'[16] However, there is no evidence that providing a more expensive primary care system has any effect on hospital referral, and it may indeed work conversely to increase requests for more specialised investigations and treatment.

The inability of central government to exert any meaningful control over the medical profession has been reflected ever since the inception of the NHS in the maldistribution of doctors throughout the country. The failure of the positive and negative incentive schemes has been documented,[17] and it appears unjustified optimism for the 1976 consultative document to state that one of its main objectives for primary care is to 'remedy persistent shortages of personnel in localities where they occur, by encouraging a better distribution of manpower '[18] without any indication as to how this might be achieved in practice. Similar problems of maldistribution and ineffective controls are mentioned in the document's discussion of general dental services.[19]

Local Authority Decision-Making

The interface between the National Health Service and Personal Social Service facilities in many ways reflects the problems encountered more generally between all central and local government services. This dichotomy leads to a highly complicated network of services with complex finance and control mechanisms. The recent Layfield Committee was unable to make any firm proposals to simplify this relationship and suggested a range of alternatives involving greater or lesser control over local government standards and financial arrangements.[20] Most local authority services are not subject to direct control from central government, and in the case of the social service facilities, after various statutory requirements have been met, the DHSS is unable to influence directly how the local authorities arrange their contribution to the caring services.

Indirect influence is exerted by the publication of various norms and guidelines and through financial manipulation of the rate support grant and cash limit system. Central government can affect local government commitments by the introduction of new statutory machinery, e.g., the Children and Young Persons Act, the Chronically Sick and Disabled Persons Act.

Local government social services have, therefore, been even more unevenly distributed than NHS services, reflecting to some degree local needs, and also dependent on the individual local authority's priorities between the various services it provides (housing, education, etc.) and its commitment to finance a portion of this expenditure from local rate collection. This uneven distribution is shown in Table 2.7.

Table 2.7.   Services in Non-Metropolitan County Authority Social Service Departments

	Highest	Lowest
Total expenditure on social services per 1,000 population	£14,932 Avon	£8,586 Salop
No. of fieldwork staff per 1,000 population	0.61 Bedford	0.26 Buckingham
Expenditure on elderly per 1,000, 65+ years	£28,809 Bedford	£14,066 Isle of Wight
Expenditure on day care for the elderly per 1,000, 65+ years	£2,323 Humberside	0 several authorities
Meals on Wheels per 1,000, 65+ years	£9,548 Cleveland	£1,681 Isle of Wight

Source: Social Services Statistics 1975/6 Estimate Provision, *County Councils Gazette,* Sept. (1975), p.163.

The problems of distribution of power have to be viewed against the present background of a very unfavourable financial climate for local authority expenditure. The Public Expenditure White Paper stated that no increase in the total of local authority current expenditure could be expected in the next few years.[21] The suggested overall growth rate of current expenditure on social services of 2.9 per cent per year[22] on which all the local authority commitments (such as the growth of domiciliary services, etc.) depend is in turn dependent on a range of conditions, none of which are under the control of the DHSS. The conditions include local authority manpower considerations, the balance between capital and current expenditure, the balance of priorities between various local authority services and the revenue implications of recent capital expenditure as well as financial provision for recent statutory provision. In addition, many local authorities are starting from a base of services that is extremely underdeveloped and poorly distributed and will feel unable to meet the requirements suggested for the provision of services in the consultative document.

A survey of social service departments showed that in their projected budgets for 1976/7 many authorities were cutting back exactly those services selected for priority in the consultative document.[23] Somerset reduced home-help hours and meals-on-wheels and cut provision for aids and adaptations for the disabled; Surrey reduced day-care provision, closed a day-care centre for the mentally ill and increased meals-on-wheels charges. Dorset cut to two hours per week per case their home-help service. Norfolk Country Council cut all capital developments, left one home for the elderly complete but unopened, doubled the price charged for meals-on-wheels, transferred a new hostel from psychiatric rehabilitation to a home for adolescents.[24] The policy planning sub-committee stated:

> People in Norfolk will need to understand that it will be harder to get help from the domestic service, harder to obtain a place in an old people's home, and it will not be possible to contemplate a single addition to the capital programme of any consequence until well after 1980.[25]

This is not to pass judgement on the relationship between the local authorities and central government, but simply to suggest that without resolution of the problems apparently inherent in the relationship, the implementation of the proposed priorities will in some areas remain far from the ideal development of services proposed in the consultative document.

It is also possible to forecast very similar developments in the practical application of the joint funding arrangements. Under this arrangement, NHS money can be used to finance certain local authority social service provisions that might relieve pressure on NHS facilities — rehabilitation facilities for psychiatric patients, etc.[26] Decisions for the use of this arrangement lie outside the control of the DHSS, and less progressive authorities might well resist the short-term benefits of the funding because after five years the financial burden will revert to the local authority again. Thus it might well come about that the joint funding will be taken up only by those local authorities that are relatively progressive and have already gone some way towards implementing the policies now made explicit in the consultative document.

Decision-Making and the Forces of Reaction

The establishment of such broad guidelines and general policy commitments will bring the DHSS under direct attack from those who feel that they have not been awarded the priority they deserve. It is clear from this document that the DHSS feels that in the past the general acute and maternity services have enjoyed a growth rate that is greater than they should command in the future. The broad plan is to restrict the growth of general and acute hospital services to 1.2 per cent per year and actually reduce the expenditure on maternity services by 2 per cent per year. It is evident that the implementation of these decisions will be resisted by those involved in these sectors. However, the reason why these particular sectors have in the past enjoyed a disproportionate advantage over the other sectors is precisely because of their immense power. This power will continue to be exerted against exactly those policies that will tend to produce equity between the sectors of the service in the way advocated.

The bias of the majority of the medical profession towards technological intervention is extensively documented elsewhere in this study. It is possible to trace this focus throughout the training that medical students receive, and it is reflected in their career choice on qualification. The major decision-making bodies of the profession are dominated by consultants representing the acute specialties, and their power is reflected in the present distribution of resources throughout the NHS.

It therefore came as no surprise that the present consultative document has been violently attacked by the profession in an editorial

in the *British Medical Journal* as 'A Policy of Despair'. In rejecting the
proposals of the DHSS, the editorial advocates increased spending on
acute hospital buildings, renal dialysis, renal transplantation and
EMI scanning equipment and pleads for the contribution of medical
technology to the treatment of coronary thrombosis, stroke, lung,
bowel and breast cancers, degenerative arthritis etc. Amazingly the
editorial comments: 'By putting people before buildings and by giving
practical expression to public sympathy for the old and the handicapped
Mrs Castle has, perhaps, allowed sentiment to overrule intellect.'[27]
The British Medical Association also joined the Royal College of
Obstetricians and Gynaecologists in advocating increased spending on
the technological components of maternity care.[28] Many of the points
that were specifically made to support their claims for increased
technological intervention have been firmly rejected by a great deal of
objective medical evidence.[29]

The Internal Dynamics of the Administration

Within the NHS administration itself there is an imperfect relationship
between the central guidelines and what actually happens at more
peripheral levels of the system. At local level there may be good reasons
why certain general guidelines cannot be followed.[30] Imperfections in
the relationship between the various tiers of the management have
recently been highlighted by the 1976 report from the team of regional
chairmen, who were highly critical of much of the organisation and
workings of the central DHSS.[31] In addition, it would be wrong to
assume that the entire management and administration of the NHS can
be considered as a single entity sharing one set of values or aspirations.
This is particularly true of the different approaches that are often
apparent between the professional managers at various levels and their
political masters within the government. Similarly at the lowest level of
management there are often tremendous tensions between the members
of district management teams drawn from various professional groups
to arrive at consensus decisions which may well not be in the interest
of their particular professional group.[32]

All these internal dynamics within the administration itself will
make rational, centrally conceived policies difficult, or even impossible
to implement in practice, yet none were mentioned in the discussion
document on priorities within the NHS.

The criticism against the administration is thus not that it is over-
manned or too expensive, but that it does not consult on the most
important issues with the people for whom services are actually

intended. Although a consultative document on priorities has been
produced, it fails to consult on the relationships of power within the
NHS, and Chapter 7 shows that the administration does not match its
rhetoric with meaningful transfers of resources for the future.

The Administration and Consultation with Community Health Councils

This failure of the administration to attempt meaningful consultation at
a national level is also apparent at local levels. Since reorganisation,
community health councils (CHCs) have been established to 'provide a
new means of representing the local community's interests in the health
service to those responsible for managing them'; moreover, 'the relevant
Area Authority has a duty to consult the CHC on any substantial
development of the health services in the council's district.'[33]

Detailed observation shows that consultation with CHCs at a local
level can be almost totally lacking in any real meaning.

In July 1976 the Norwich District Management Team submitted
their own consultative document, styled the Norwich District Plan,[34]
for the approval of the local community health council. The following
notes were written in response to this consultative document and
illustrate well that the administration of the NHS locally does not
take consultation with the local community, here represented by the
CHC, in any way seriously.

1. The Method of Consultation

The timing of the consultation and the speed expected for reply does
not give confidence that the document is concerned to produce
meaningful consultation. It was presented for discussion at the 13 July
meeting of the CHC, the deadline for reply being the beginning of
August. Unfortunately, there is no CHC meeting in August, and the
CHC agenda was already too full to discuss it at any length at the July
meeting.

No offer was made that the members of the District Management
Team should present the document in person to the CHC and explain
in detail the implications of the proposals.

Questions: Does this speedy consultation imply that, unless there are
specific objections, the CHC has given blanket approval for all the plans
in the document, including the closure of all the units singled out for
this treatment in the document?

Who else is being consulted about this document? Presumably the
staff-side implications are being dealt with, but is the consultation with

them of a similar cursory nature? Was their consultation also in the middle of the holiday period?

Should the CHCs find out what the staff-side implications of the plans are with regard to employment, conditions, etc., and use the expert knowledge of trades union representatives as well as the opinions of the District Management Team before making any response to the document?

2. The Style of Consultation

Virtually no new figures are presented in the document on the financial implications of any of the proposals. It is therefore difficult, or impossible, really to make sensible comments about the proposals. It appears that the majority of NHS decisions are presently made on financial grounds, rather than with the objective of providing the best services for the patients. However, without any indication of the costs or savings involved in the various proposals, it is difficult to comment on the planning being undertaken.

The entire document is very vague indeed, and it appears to present schemes for almost any combination of events, rather than a single plan of detailed proposals for CHC comment or approval. To take an example: it would appear that the District Management Team might or might not try to convert the David Rice Hospital for use as an in-patient and/or out-patient psychiatric hospital for children. . .the space possibly produced at the Bethel Hospital might then be used for geriatric or psychiatric day hospitals, or for office accommodation. . .[35]

Questions: What is the actual plan for consultation? How and when will the real decisions be taken, and by whom? Does CHC acquiescence at this stage imply that any of the possibilities are OK with the community?

Is the entire planning exercise represented in this document simply rationalisation for economic reasons alone? Almost no mention is made of service to the patient, access for relatives, etc.

3. The Content of the Consultation

It would appear that the document mirrors the importance attached relatively to the hospital and community services. In its forty pages there is only one mention of the community health services. This does not, in fact, give any details of plans for the future of community services, but concerns itself with the barest administrative details of the service and the purchase of health centre sites. This section states:

'Discussions are also taking place to see what other developments should occur during the next 5 to 10 years in the Community Health Services.'[36]

With whom are these discussions and can the CHC join in?

Because of the lack of hard data mentioned previously, it is almost impossible to compare the priorities that are proposed in this district plan with the major DHSS document, *Priorities for Health and Personal Social Services.* There has been no attempt to link together the general DHSS guides with these specific district plans. The only reference comes in the section on maternity services for Drayton Hall, which says that the DHSS guidelines will not be adhered to.[37]

Questions: The document has not attempted to follow the same pattern as the DHSS guidelines and introduce an analysis by client groups. The one mention of DHSS guidelines specifically rejects them. What are the implications in growth terms for the elderly, the mentally handicapped, etc., in the district?

What are the plans for the community health services? Or does the complete absence of plans in this document mean that once again the community services are only considered last?

Joint Planning and Joint Funding. The prospect of joint funding and joint planning with local authority social services as in DHSS Circular HC(76)18 has been warmly welcomed by the CHC. The hope is that this arrangement will eradicate some of the gaps in the present services. Unfortunately, this first planning document from the District Management Team since the production of this important DHSS circular makes no mention at all of joint planning.

Have the social services nothing to say about the plans? Will they be consulted, and, if so, will it be in the same style as the consultation with the CHC and without access to the full figures? Is this joint planning now taking place at area level? If so, who represents the voice of the consumer at this level, and how?

The joint funding projects mentioned in the document are for Hellesdon Psychiatric Day Hospital and Eaton Grange Day Hospital. No indication is given, however, of the acceptability of these schemes to the Norfolk County Council. What will happen to the patients if the local authority will not join in these schemes and do not want to accept the financial burden for the projects after five years?

Community Hospitals. The plans mention that community hospitals might be considered for Dereham, Wayland, North Walsham, Kelling, and Cromer. What does this actually mean? In what way would community hospitals be different from the facilities that are already provided on these sites? Would community hospitals have more facilities, or less, or just have a change of name for the same thing? What would be the financial implications of the development of these community hospitals?

Question: Does the development of community hospitals really depend on more guidance from the DHSS, or should the District Management Team submit a strong positive plan to introduce these hospitals on the sites mentioned for the approval of the DHSS? What exactly is the next step?

4. The Mood of the Consultation

The entire mood of the document is one of contraction, conservatism, and gloom. The present financial stringency could be used by management at all levels to review the entire shape of the NHS and the effectiveness of its efforts. It does not have to mean simple contraction, into the situation where the service is only able to do less of the same. It is almost certain that the time of a financial boom is quite a long way in the future. Does this mean that the people in need have to wait for that time until satisfactory services can be provided?

The development of preventive health measures, community services, joint planning and co-ordination of the services are more important than ever now, and the scarcity of resources should be taken as a positive opportunity to develop a service better equipped for the needs of the people in the district.

Unfortunately, this consultative document fails to consult, and fails to mention any of these positive measures.

Health Service Commissioner: There is additional evidence from the reports of the Health Service Commissioner that the administration of the NHS can be lacking in quality in its dealings with the community. It is the Health Service Commissioner's task to investigate complaints made by members of the public against the administration of the NHS. In his first year (1974/5) he upheld 53 per cent (68) of these complaints, and his reports detail many incidents in which the administration was found to be lacking in its actions and on which he has 'invited the authority to review administrative practices and procedures'.[38]

Notes and References

1. Department of Health and Social Security, *Statistics for Health and Personal Social Services* (HMSO, London, 1975).
2. Department of Treasury, *Public Expenditure to 1975/6,* Cmnd. 4829 (HMSO, London, 1971).
3. K. Barnard and C. Ham, 'The Reallocation of Resources', *Lancet* (1976), vol.1, p.1399.
4. Department of Health and Social Security, *Priorities for Health and Personal Social Services* (HMSO, London, 1976).
5. Ibid., para.2.1.
6. *Report of Committee of Inquiry into the Pay and Related Conditions of Service of Nurses and Midwives* (Chairman: Lord Halsbury) (HMSO, London, 1974).
7. *Doctors' and Dentists' Remuneration, Fifth Report* (Chairman: Sir Ernest Woodroofe), Cmnd. 6032 (HMSO, London, 1975).
8. These figures come from a speech by David Owen to the Medical Practitioners' Union, 6 December 1975.
9. DHSS, *Priorities,* para.2.1.
10. R.F.L. Logan, *The Dynamics of Medical Care,* Memo. No.14 (London School of Hygiene and Tropical Medicine, 1972).
11. For a summary of some of this evidence see DHSS, *Priorities,* Appendix A.
12. See, for instance, Editorial, *British Medical Journal (BMJ)* (1974), vol.1, p.255.
13. *Report of Committee of Inquiry into the Regulation of the Medical Profession* (Chairman: Dr A.W. Merrison), Cmnd.6018 (HMSO, London, 1975).
14. DHSS, *Priorities,* para. 4.20.
15. DHSS, *Priorities,* para. 3.5.
16. Ibid.
17. R.J. Butler, *Family Doctors and Public Policy* (Routledge and Kegan Paul, London, 1973).
18. DHSS, *Priorities,* para. 3.6.
19. DHSS, *Priorities,* para. 3.14.
20. *Local Government Finance: A Report of the Committee of Inquiry,* Cmnd. 6453 (HMSO, London, 1976).
21. Public Expenditure White Paper, Cmnd. 6393 (HMSO, London, 1976) pp.92-6.
22. DHSS, *Priorities,* para. 10.8.
23. Published by British Association of Social Workers, 17 December 1975. Available from BASW, 16 Kent Street, Birmingham B5 6RD.
24. Norfolk County Council, Minutes of the Full Council, 25 October 1975.
25. Norfolk County Council, Minutes of Social Services Committee, 22 December 1975. For fuller criticism of the decisions taken by the Social Services Department at this time, see Child Poverty Action Group special newsletter, 'Social Services in Norfolk'. Available from Norwich CPAG, 8 Winter Road, Norwich.
26. DHSS Circular HC (76) 18 (DHSS, 1976).
27. 'A Policy of Despair', Editorial, *BMJ* (1976), vol.1, p.787.
28. Royal College of Obstetricians and Gynaecologists, press statement, 7 June 1976.
29. Almost all the specific claims made in the campaign to defend increased spending on obstetric care, etc., have been disputed, and none stand up well to rigorous scientific evaluation. See H. Campbell *et al., BMJ* (1976), vol.1, p.1013; P. Kirk, *BMJ* (1976), vol.1, p.1014.

30. B. Waitkin, *Themes in Health Care Planning* (University of Manchester, 1976); A. Mills and J. Reynolds, 'Centre-Periphery: Can Guidelines Bridge the Gap?', *Hospital and Health Services Review* (1977), vol.73, no.2, p.50.

31. 'Regional Chairmen's Enquiry into the Working of the DHSS in Relation to Regional Health Authorities', May 1976. Available from M.J. Fairey, NE Thames Authority.

32. F. Pethybridge, 'Multidisciplinary Management and Decision-Making in the Reorganized NHS', *Hospital and Health Services Review* (1976), vol.72, no.3, p.77; J. Lewis, 'Reorganization: The First Year, View from the Districts', *BMJ* (1976), vol.2, p.22.

33. DHSS Circular HRC (74) 4 (DHSS, 1974).

34. Norwich District Management Team, 'Norwich District Plan' (unpublished, July 1976).

35. Ibid., p.16.

36. Ibid., p.34.

37. Ibid., p.18.

38. House of Commons Papers, *First Report of the Health Service* Commissioner, No.407, Session 1974-5 (HMSO, London, 1975); No.528, Session 1975-6 (HMSO, London, 1976); No.322, Session 1976-7 (HMSO, London, 1977).

3 THE MEDICAL PROFESSION

The medical profession is the second group within the health service that has enormous power and is responsible, with the administration, for the shape and future direction that the health services take. The medical profession, however, in pursuing its own aims, is not necessarily acting in the best interests of the health service, or the majority of the community. This is illustrated below by four sets of considerations: (1) insistence on total autonomy; (2) the ineffectiveness of sanctions against the profession; (3) the technological orientation of current medical practice; (4) the continuance of private practice within the NHS and aggressive wage bargaining.

Total Professional Autonomy

The medical profession is vociferously insistent on the maintenance of total autonomy. However, this is not without its financial cost to the health service and the general community. The argument has been well rehearsed recently, and several studies have shown that the immense variations between the practices of individual doctors and the continued use of a great many interventions without proven effectiveness is very expensive to the health service.[1]

David Owen has recently calculated that each consultant, on average, spends £250,000 annually, and that each general practitioner controls annual resources worth £25,000.[2]

It would appear to be obvious that major savings could be made comparatively simply by the introduction of a system of medical audit. The savings made through the rational prescription of pharmaceuticals, and by restriction of medical intervention to procedures of proven effectiveness, would release money for the development of innovatory services and for the support of those services presently starved of funds. The real debate remains as to whether this audit should be performed by the administration or by the medical profession itself in order to maintain its autonomy.

The case for rational prescribing would appear unanswerable in terms of patient care. The increasing complexity and diversity of medicines almost continually introduced onto the market has led to enormous difficulties for medical practitioners both in hospital and in general practice. The very large numbers of similar medicines sold under different brand names, which often obscure pharmacological properties, has led to an increasing incidence of drug interactions and morbidity and mortality from prescribed medicines.

Each year nearly 3,000 people die in England and Wales as a result of drug overdosage and therapeutic misadventure.[3] Adverse reactions to medicines account for 5 per cent of admissions to hospital medical wards, and between 10 per cent and 15 per cent of patients suffer an adverse reaction of one type or another during admission.[4]

Many of the medicines presently available for prescribing have no proven efficacy. As part of the Sainsbury Committee enquiry into the relationship of the pharmaceutical industry with the NHS, two independent teams of experts assessed the therapeutic value of the 2,657 proprietary preparations available on NHS prescription. Of the 84 per cent of the preparations on which the two panels were in complete agreement, 35 per cent were considered to be *undesirable* for one or several reasons.[5]

A year after the NHS began (1949), Britain's drug bill was £39 million; in 1974 it had risen to £327 million.[6]

From 1972/3 to 1973/4 the growth rate of the hospital drugs bill was greater than the growth rate of any other sector of the budget — 23 per cent, as Table 3.1 shows.

A comparable acceleration has also been apparent in the bill for family practitioner pharmaceutical services, which had an annual growth rate of 13 per cent in 1971/2, 11 per cent in 1972/3, and 17 per cent in 1973/4.[7] The DHSS consultative document *Priorities* states that the pharmaceutical services cost £310 million,[8] which represents 43 per cent of the total cost of all primary care services of £720 million.

It is quite clear that the majority of medicines presently prescribed are not utilised for life-saving therapeutic interventions, but represent 'the relentless march of the psychotropic drug juggernaut'.[9]

The cost-effectiveness of the various drug therapies that are available on prescription seems to have received scant attention. For each of the medicines prescribed, there are frequently equally effective, but cheaper, preparations available. In many cases, the same medicine is available on the market at several different prices marketed by different manufacturers. One example of this has been documented in the price of corticosteroid preparations, although similar examples could be cited in every other group of drugs:

I know of no evidence that any oral preparation of corticosteroid is superior to prednisolone for the treatment of conditions such as

Table 3.1.   Growth Rate of Expenditure in Various NHS Sectors 1972/3 to 1973/4

Sector	% growth rate
Total hospital current (revenue) expenditure	16
Salaries and wages:	
Medical and dental	11
Nursing	13
Other	19
Provisions	21
Staff uniforms and patients' clothing	17
Drugs	23
Dressings	17
Medical and surgical appliances and equipment	17
General·services	11
Maintenance of buildings, plant, and grounds	13
Domestic repairs	21
Blood transfusion, mass radiography, etc.	15
Other expenditure	13
Central administration	21

Source: DHSS, *Health and Personal Social Service Statistics for England* (HMSO, London, 1976).

Table 3.2.   Annual Growth in Hospitals' Drugs Bill 1970/1 to 1973/4

	1970/1 to 1971/2	1971/2 to 1972/3	1972/3 to 1973/4
% annual growth	13	13	23

Source: DHSS, *Health and Personal Social Service Statistics for England* (HMSO, London, 1976).

rheumatoid arthritis and asthma. Prednisolone obtained from the least expensive source costs less than 30p per 100 5 mg tablets (basic NHS price), but most manufacturers charge 42p for the same quantity of their branded product, and one firm charges as much as 94p. Equivalent amounts of drugs such as bethamethasone (85p), dexamethasone (£2.82), and triamcinolone £4.70) are even more expensive, and methylprednisolone (£5.14) is the most expensive of all.[10]

Table 3.3. Number of NHS Prescriptions in 1974 by Therapeutic
            Category

Therapeutic category	Numbers of prescriptions
Tranquillisers and hypnotics	38,864,000
Antipyretic analgesics	18,017,000
Penicillins	17,689,000
Expectorants and cough suppressants	17,112,000
Diuretics	11,401,000
Tetracyclines	10,236,000
Corticosteroid preparations acting on the skin	10,087,000
Preparations used in rheumatic diseases	9,930,000
Antacids and antispasmodics	9,440,000

Source: DHSS, *Health and Personal Social Service Statistics for England* (HMSO, London, 1976).

There is a range of alternatives that could be implemented to rationalise both the safety and cost of prescribed medicines. These might include:

(1) The introduction of a restricted list of medicines that could be prescribed by doctors at various levels of the NHS.[11] Thus general practitioners might not have automatic access to the entire range of complex and costly drugs, while some hospital consultants would continue to be able to prescribe the entire range.

(2) Testing medicines on the approved lists for efficacy as well as safety. In other words, drugs that do not work could no longer be prescribed on the NHS.[12]

(3) Ensuring the continuing education of doctors with regard to pharmaceutical matters. The above measures might make such education simpler and more effective. At present doctors rely on the promotional efforts of the manufacturers to inform them of the pharmaceutical properties of the marketed drugs. This method leads to undervaluation of the benefits of cost-effective prescribing.

(4) Requiring that the writing of prescriptions be done using generic (pharmaceutically active) names rather than brand names. This would help in the education of doctors and would also ensure that the NHS could supply the cheapest available product. If doctors wanted to specify a particular brand to be used, then they could retain the right to indicate this in brackets by the side of the generic name.[13]

These suggestions are restricted to the rational prescription of medicines and have not included any direct proposals for alterations in the structure of the drug industry itself (nationalisation, etc.). This matter in itself is of importance to the NHS and is receiving attention elsewhere.[14]

The case for more rational prescription of medicines would appear unanswerable, and the reasons why none of these measures has so far been introduced lies in the realms of the political and financial interests of the medical profession and multinational pharmaceutical industry, rather than in the arena of rational debate.

Absence of Sanctions

The lack of sanctions against the medical profession has been well documented in the case of complaints against general practitioners[15] and also with regard to complaints against members of the medical profession working in hospitals.[16] The Health Service Commissioner has no jurisdiction over questions involving the clinical judgement of doctors,[17] and the recent Merrison Committee, which was established to 'consider what changes need to be made in the existing provisions for the regulation of the medical profession', advocated a strengthening, rather than a revision, of the concept of complete medical autonomy. The committee suggested that 'the medical profession should be largely self-regulated, and should be regulated by an independent body'. The suggested 'independent body' (the General Medical Council, or GMC) should be composed of 98 members — 88 of whom should be members of the medical profession.[18]

The interests of the general public appear protected only when gross infringements have taken place. The GMC can strike doctors from the medical register and prevent them from practising medicine in this country. However, the Merrison Committee suggested that the scope of the GMC should be restricted to those cases which represent a 'general public risk' and think 'the GMC should take care to explain why it cannot look into every action by a doctor brought to its notice, and that it must be concerned only with matters which question the continuance of a doctor's registration.'.

Technological Orientation

The medical profession remains largely orientated towards the technological components of medical practice. Medical education focuses on the advanced technological specialties; medical students thus aspire to join the specialties which attract great kudos and a much increased share of health service resources.

A survey of 25 medical schools found that only 7 schools gave six or more hours to the subject of occupational medicine, and 10 schools (including 8 in London) neglected the subject altogether.[19] Another survey showed that even four years after the Royal Commission on Medical Education had recommended the establishment of departments of community medicine, only four of the twelve London medical schools had done so.[20] Similar gaps exist in the teaching of geriatrics and even in the training for primary care. The emphasis on technological specialities is reflected in the career preferences of medical students (See Table 3.4.)[21]

The technological specialties also receive the bulk of the merit awards. Of the specialists in thoracic surgery, 73 per cent receive merit awards; 70 per cent of those in cardiology, 63 per cent of those in neurosurgery — while only 25 per cent of specialists in mental health, 23 per cent in geriatrics, and less than 3 per cent in community medicine receive these awards.[22]

British-born and British-trained doctors fill the majority of consultant posts in the favoured technological specialties, while those from abroad are only able to reach consultancies in the less technological specialties. In 1972, 25 per cent of consultants and 61 per cent of senior registrars were trained overseas; however, only 9 per cent of consultants and 12 per cent of senior registrars in the specialty of

Table 3.4. Career Preferences of Medical Students: First Choices

Career choice	Royal Commission	Manchester & Sheffield Enquiry	
	1968 %	1971 %	1972 %
Medicine	26.5	24.0	23.8
Surgery	17.8	19.9	13.5
Obstetrics and gynaecology	12.4	5.5	4.0
General practice	23.5	32.2	46.8
Psychiatry	5.2	1.4	2.4
Community medicine	1.6	2.0	1.6
Pathology	2.1	3.4	4.7
Anaesthetics	2.0	8.2	3.2
Radiology	0.8	0.7	—
Other	8.1	2.7	—

Source: C. McLaughlin, 'Career Preferences', *Lancet* (1974), vol.1, p.870.

general medicine were from overseas. Between 1969 and 1972, 9 per cent of new consultant posts in general surgery and 17 per cent of new posts in general medicine went to doctors trained overseas, while 50 per cent of consultant posts in geriatrics and 71 per cent in venereology were awarded to this group.[23]

The effects of this concentration by the medical profession on highly advanced technological medicine are discussed in Chapter 4. The bulk of health services resources are concentrated in this sector to the detriment of the majority of patients suffering from the more common complaints of psychiatric illness or the complications of old age. This focus also detracts from the practice of, and the distribution of resources to, the preventive services.

Private Practice within the NHS

The power of the medical profession is exhibited not only in its control over decision-making, but also by its ability to continue to practise private medicine within the National Health Service. The continuance of this practice is only of advantage to the members of the profession who do private work (e.g., 88 per cent of general surgeons) and to the small numbers of fortunate people who can afford private fees or who belong to various group insurance schemes.

The advantage to the medical profession is considerable. An example was given by a consultant surgeon in the fourth report of the government expenditure committee on National Health Service facilities for private patients:

> I am giving up £800 per year (2/11 of NHS salary). I am doing one patient a week who brings me in approximately £75 to £100 per week for 52 weeks of the year, something like £5,000. I have expenses admittedly, but I am giving up £800 and getting £5,000.[24]

In 1974, £8,780,000 was paid by medical insurance schemes alone to consultant surgeons.[25]

The advantage to private patients in terms of waiting time for routine operations is very considerable. The Royal College of Nursing did a survey of 84 centres, and the results were published in the Government report quoted above. (See Table 3.5.)

The NHS does not gain from maintaining private pay beds within the service. The income received from pay beds is quite small and does not cover the cost of maintaining these beds. (See Table 3.6.)

Some simple arithmetic shows that this income did not cover the

Table 3.5.   Waiting Times for Operations

Operation	Length of Waiting Time	
	Private	NHS
Hysterectomy	2 weeks	4 months
Vasectomy	2 weeks	2 years
Gynae operations	1 week	12 months
Cataract	2 weeks	over 1 month
Tonsilectomy	2 weeks	18 months

Source: NHS, *Facilities for Private Patients,* Fourth Report of the Expenditure Committee, Session 1971-72 (HMSO, London, 1972).

Table 3.6.   Annual Income to NHS from Pay Beds

Year	Income £
1972-3	11,951,911
1973-4	13,702,967
1974-5	15,000,000 (provisional)

Source: House of Commons Written Answer, 25 November 1975.

costs involved. In 1972 there were 4,923 pay beds; each cost approximately £90 to maintain each week. This totals £23.4 million, while the income from pay beds during that year was only £11.9 million. Since then the income from pay beds has risen, but so has the cost of providing these facilities in NHS hospitals.

Calculations can also be made for individual hospitals. In 1973-4, the NHS income from the 37 private pay beds at the Norfolk and Norwich Hospital was £115,490. However, these beds each cost about £90 each week to maintain, so the annual running costs were at least £173,160.[26]

In addition, the capital costs involved are very considerable. Each bed in a district general hospital represents a capital outlay of approximately £20,000, so the NHS capital currently tied up in private beds is over £100 million.

The bed occupancy rate for pay beds is very low. In 1974, the 4,574 authorised pay beds had an average daily occupancy rate of 2,245 (under 50 per cent), compared with the average rate of over 80 per cent for all other NHS beds.[27]

Aggressive Wage Bargaining

The medical profession has recently become very aggressive regarding its wage bargaining position and has, on several occasions, either gone on strike or threatened strike action in order to further its own interests. Without going into details regarding the rates of remuneration of each grade of hospital doctor or of doctors in general practice, the medical profession does apparently continue to enjoy a very high standard of living. The full-time salary scale of consultants per annum in 1975 was between £7,536 and £10,689, and the average for all general practitioners was £8,485 (excluding the additional remuneration from the contraceptive services).[28] The most junior hospital doctor, after qualification but before registration (usually in his or her early twenties), earns a basic wage just below the national average total income, and take-home pay at this most junior level is well above the average national income.

Increases in the pay of doctors come out of the total health service budget, and it is evident that higher levels of remuneration enjoyed by the medical profession will be at the expense of other groups of employees or at the expense of services for patients.

Poorly endowed regions have recently been allocated additional 'development funds' in order to bring their services more in line with national averages. The East Anglian Region is one of the poorest regions, and development funds have been allocated to the areas within it. However, a large proportion of the money given to the Norfolk Area Health Authority to improve services has gone for the increased overtime payments of the junior hospital staff, and has not therefore been available to improve services in the area.[29]

In the Cambridgeshire area, for instance, over 50 per cent of the available 'development' money was spent on the costs of the new junior hospital doctors' contract. The total expenditure for the whole region amounts to almost £500,000 which would have surely been money intended for the improvement of actual services for patients in the region.

Summary

This chapter on the medical profession has given examples of the power of the medical profession as a group, and has given instances where the interests of the profession are not necessarily the same as the interests of the entire community. Possibly the most important point to emerge is the documenting of the decision-making power of the profession. In no sense are the decisions of the profession made in partnership with the administration or, more particularly, with any decision-making apparatus within the community. This does not imply that the decisions made by the profession are never in the interest of the community, but that they are always taken on a unilateral basis.[30]

The following chapters describe in detail the effects of this sort of decision-making, and the effects of the power dynamic between the government/administration and the medical profession.

This is not to suggest that the medical profession should surrender all its power, status and autonomy, but simply that it should consider a new sort of relationship with the community it purports to serve, whereby decision-making is a matter of co-operation rather than unilateral action. This relationship would naturally extend to the level of individual doctors' dealings with individual members of the community. It does seem an anachronism for the medical profession to keep to itself all knowledge about disease processes, etc., at the same time as it bemoans the fact that many consultations are apparently for trivial reasons. Certainly the task of the medical profession in the future should include the specialised treatment of those who have become ill; but above all, it should increasingly be orientated to teaching the community how to stay healthy and how to cope with simple ailments as they arise.

Notes and References

1. A.L. Cochrane, *Effectiveness and Efficiency* (Nuffield Provincial Hospitals Trust, London, 1971). See also DHSS, *Priorities for Health and Personal Social Services* (HMSO, London, 1976), Appendix A.
2. David Owen, 'The NHS and Public Expenditure', *New Statesman*, 23 April 1976, p.532.
3. Registrar General, *Annual Statistics for Deaths in England and Wales 1973* (HMSO, London, 1975). Quoted in *BMJ*, 'Editorial', (1976), vol.1, p.413.
4. O.L. Wade, *Adverse Reactions to Drugs* (Heinemann, London, 1970).
5. *Report of the Committee of Inquiry into the Relationship of the Pharmaceutical Industry with the National Health Service 1965-7* (Sainsbury Committee), Cmnd. 3410 (HMSO, London, 1967).
6. 'NHS Drug Costs', *Lancet* (1976), vol.1., p.921.
7. DHSS, *Health and Personal Social Service Statistics for England* (HMSO, London, 1975).
8. DHSS, *Priorities for Health and Personal Social Services in England* (HMSO, London, 1976), para. 3.1.
9. W.H. Trethowan, 'Pills for Personal Problems', *BMJ* (1975), vol.2, p.749.
10. L.W.B. Grant, 'Cost of Drugs', *BMJ* (1973), vol.1, p.416.
11. N. Olsen, 'Restricted Drugs List of NHS Drugs?', *BMJ* (1974), vol.2, p.273.

12. This has already been standard practice under the U.S. Food and Drug Administration for many years.
13. Many of these ideas have been tried in several 'developing' nations. For a report of the situation in Sri Lanka, see S.A. Wickremasinghe and S. Bibile, 'Pharmaceuticals Management in Ceylon', *BMJ* (1971), vol.2, p.757; and for an excellent article on cost effectiveness and the prescription of medicines in the developing world, see A.N.P. Speight, 'Cost Effectiveness and Drug Therapy', *Tropical Doctor,* April 1975, p.89.
14. T.D. Heller, *Poor Health, Rich Profits* (Spokesman Books, Nottingham, 1977). See also *The Pharmaceutical Industry* (The Labour Party, London, 1976); 'Nationalisation and the Pharmaceutical Industry', *Lancet* (1976), vol.1, p.1196; 'Politics and Pharmaceuticals', *BMJ* (1976), vol.1, p.1105; 'Towards Better Prescribing', *Lancet* (1976), vol.1, p.1249.
15. R. Klein, *Complaints against Doctors* (Charles Knight, London, 1973).
16. M. Stacey, 'Consumer Complaints in the British NHS', *Social Science and Medicine* (1974), vol.8, p.429.
17. House of Commons Paper, *First Report of the Health Service Commissioner,* No.407, Session 1974-5 (HMSO, London, 1975).
18. *Report of the Committee of Inquiry into the Regulation of the Medical Profession* (Chairman: Dr. A.W. Merrison), Cmnd. 6018 (HMSO, London, 1975).
19. H.A. Waldron, 'Undergraduate Training in Occupational Medicine', *Lancet* (1974), vol.2, p.277.
20. Editorial, 'Who's for Community Medicine?', *Lancet* (1972), vol.2, p.1297.
21. C. McLaughlin, 'Career Preferences', *Lancet* (1974), vol.1, p.870.
22. DHSS, *Annual Report* (HMSO, London, 1974).
23. G.I.B. Da Costa, 'The Overseas Doctor and the Hospital Service', *Consultant* (1974), vol.21, p.10; see also *Doctors from Overseas: A case for consultation* (Community Relations Commission, London, 1976).
24. *NHS Facilities for Private Patients,* Fourth Report of the Expenditure Committee, No.172, Session 1971-2 (HMSO, London, 1972).
25. 'UK Private Medical Care. Provident Scheme Statistics 1974' (Lee Donaldson Associates, London).
26. Norfolk Area Health Authority, *Financial Accounts 1975.*
27. House of Commons Written Answer, 20 January 1976.
28. House of Commons Written Answer, 24 March 1976.
29. Norfolk Area Health Authority, Minutes, 20 July 1976.
30. *Competence to Practise, the report of the committee of inquiry set up for the medical profession in the United Kingdom* (Committee of Inquiry into Competence to Practise, London, 1976).

4 HEALTH SERVICE DISTORTIONS

The two chapters dealing with the administration and the medical profession have given examples of the power of both these groups. The shape of the health service is determined largely by the dynamic interaction between these two groups. It is evident that the interests of these two major decision-making groups are often at variance with each other. One might suggest that at the simplest level the interests of the administration lie in striving to rationalise the service and control the power, and especially the spending potential, of the medical profession. The medical profession resists the attempts at control and protects its orientation towards technological practice. This dynamic, together with the services inherited at the inception of the NHS, has created the present distortions in the shape of the service, and also prevents these distortions from being ironed out for the benefit of the community at large.

We can examine the present distortions of the service under four separate headings: (1) patchy distribution of resources; (2) concentration on curative and institutional services at the expense of domiciliary and preventive services; (3) mismatch between needs and resources; (4) fragmentation of caring services.

Patchy Distribution of Resources

The patchy distribution of resources at regional level has been recognised since the inception of the NHS, and more recent attention has been directed towards the disparities at area level.[1] Studies of the East Anglian Region show that the variations are even greater at the level of the individual districts within the region.

The provision of all services in the East Anglian Region are well below the average provision for the other English regions. This can be shown for overall expenditure on health and social services (Table 4.1), spending on hospital services (Tables 4.2 and 4.3), and all forms of community care (Tables 4.4 and 4.5). In addition, tables are presented to show the paucity of resources in social work attachment to medical agencies (Table 4.6), psychiatric services (Table 4.7) and general practice (Table 4.8).

Table 4.1.   Expenditure per Head of Population on Health and Social
Services 1975/6

	Expenditure per head £	% diff. from England average
NHS		
England average	44.8	
East Anglia Health Authority	39.63	−11.5
Social services		
England average	14.72	
Norfolk	12.449	−15.4
Suffolk	10.01	−32
Cambs.	10.85	−26
East Anglia average	11.103	−24.6

Source: East Anglian Regional Health Authority, (i) *Revenue Allocation 1975/6;*
(ii) *Health District Profiles;* Norfolk County Council, *Report of the County
Treasurer 1975/6.* Social Service Statistics (CIPFA), Estimates 1975/6.

Table 4.2.   Hospital Services: Revenue Expenditure Per Head of
Population 1975/6

Jurisdiction	Hospital services revenue expenditure per head £	% diff. from England average
England average	36.94	−40.3
Norfolk	22.06	−40.3
Suffolk	28.10	−23.9
Cambs.	26.93	−27.1
East Anglia average	26.88	−27.2

Source: East Anglian Regional Health Authority, *Revenue Allocation 1975/6.*

Table 4.3. Provision of Hospital Resources 1972

Resource	East Anglia	England	East Anglia % difference from mean
Allocated beds per 1,000 pop.	7.8	9.0	−13.3
Unit cost per in-patient week	50.75	56.82	−10.6
Beds available per 1,000 pop.			
Medical	0.9	1.2	−25.0
Surgical	1.2	1.6	−25.0
Psychiatric	3.1	3.7	−16.2
Total hospital staff (w.t.e. per 100,000 pop.)	1,074.3	1,261.6	−14.8
Medical and dental staff	47.3	58.4	−19.0
Professional and technical staff	66.0	84.2	−21.6
Hospital nurses and midwives	450.0	521.0	−13.6

Source: Central Statistical Office, *Abstract of Regional Statistics* (HMSO, London, 1974).

Table 4.4. Facilities for community Care Provided by the NHS 1975/6

Area Health Authority	Community services £ revenue per head pop.	% difference from England average
Norfolk	2.18	−58.6
Suffolk	2.4	−54.5
Cambs.	2.08	−60.5
East Anglia average	2.3	−56.4
England average	5.27	

Source: J. Noyce, 'Regional Variations in the Allocation of Financial Resources to the Community Health Services', *Lancet* (1974), vol.1, p.554; East Anglian Regional Health Authority, *Revenue Allocation 1975/6*.

Table 4.5.   Expenditure on Various Community Social Services in
Norfolk 1976/7

£ per relevant 1,000 pop.	Norfolk	Average non-metropolitan counties	Norfolk % diff. from average
Day nurseries	1,524	3,925	−60
Pre-school playgroups	110	247	−55
Day centres and clubs	919	1,176	−22
Home helps (per 1,000 pop.)	0.70	0.83	−16
Meals	536	818	−34
Aids and adaptations	76	94	−14
Telephones	16	54	−70
Holidays	20	19	+ 5
Sheltered housing	711	958	−26

Source: Social Services Statistics (CIPFA), *Estimate Provisions 1976/7.*

Table 4.6.   Social Workers in Post and Attached to Medical Agencies, 1972

	E Anglia	England	Highest area	Lowest area	E Anglia rating	% diff. from mean
Social workers in post per million pop.	184	209	Gt. London 334	E. Midlands 174	7/9	−12
Social workers attached to med. agencies w.t.e. per million pop.	2.70	3.3	Gt. London 9.59	Yorks. & Humber 0.67	5/9	−18.2
Community medical attachments w.t.e. per million pop.	0.48	1.08	Gt. London 3.70	North 0.33	6/9	−55.5

Source: L. Ratoff *et al.,* 'Seebohm and the NHS: A survey of Medico-Social
Liaison', *BMJ* Supplement (1973), vol.2, p.51.

Table 4.7. Psychiatric Service Provision 1972

	East Anglia	England	E Anglia % difference from mean
Psychiatric beds per 1,000 pop.	3.1	3.7	−16.2
Consultants in mental illness per 1,000 pop.	1.77	1.92	− 8.0
Staff per 100 residents:			
Consultants	0.69	0.74	− 7.0
Other medical staff	1.20	1.36	−12.0
Qualified nurses	22.6	23.0	− 2.0
Psychologists	0.31	0.35	−11.0
Social workers	0.44	0.55	−20.0
Therapists	0.11	0.15	−27.0
Orderlies and domestic	7.2	8.2	−12.0

Source: DHSS, *Facilities and Services of Mental Illness Hospitals,* Statistical and Research Report Series No.8 (HMSO, London, 1974).

Table 4.8. General Practice Statistics

	Year	E Anglia average	England average	Highest region	Lowest region	E Anglia % diff. from mean
Expenditure per 1,000 pop. £	1971/2	9,446	9,609	NW Metr. 10,800	NW Metr. 8,602	−1.7
Average list size	1973	2,309	398	Yorks. 2,398	S.West	+ 3.7
% working in health centres	1975	10	14	Northern 24	Metropl. 9	−28

Source: J. R. Butler, *Family Doctors and Public Policy* (Routledge and Kegan Paul, London, 1973); Central Statistical Office, *Abstract of Regional Statistics (1974)* (HMSO, London, 1974); House of Lords, 17 December 1975, Lord Wells-Pestell.

Intraregional Distribution of Resources

Within the East Anglian Region there are enormous variations in the levels and standards of services provided both by the NHS and through local authority social services. The tables in this section illustrate the patchy nature of service provision. Table 4.9 shows the NHS revenue and capital allocation per head of population by health district, illustrates the enormous range of provision, and demonstrates that the districts that are well provided with hospital facilities also have good community services. In other words, the districts containing poor hospital services cannot compensate for this deficiency by building up domiciliary services.

Table 4.10 illustrates the staffing levels in each district, and Table 4.11 indicates the effect of the different levels of service provision on the people living in the various health districts. It can be seen that the Cinderella districts of Great Yarmouth and King's Lynn have the lowest expenditure on all aspects of health service provision and the lowest staffing levels, and that inhabitants have to wait longer for treatment, or travel outside their own district for treatment more frequently, than the people in other districts.

The distribution of local authority social service facilities within the region is shown in Table 4.1. The intra-county distribution of resources can be shown by examining the statistics prior to the 1974 reorganisation of social service departments. In Norfolk, for instance, prior to reorganisation the County Boroughs of Great Yarmouth and Norwich were administered separately from the remainder of Norfolk County. Table 4.12 shows the amazing paucity of resources in the rural areas.

Patterns of Provision of Care within Each Service

This section will examine the patterns of provision of care within the NHS and social services. It will be shown that in both services the major part of the resources is allocated to various types of acute treatment or institutional care, while preventive work takes only a small proportion of the budget of both services.

Table 4.13 illustrates the focus of attention within the health service by showing that one hospital with only 578 beds receives almost as much revenue allocation per year as the entire services for Great Yarmouth and King's Lynn, including the hospital services. The population of these two districts is over 342,000.

Table 4.14 provides a breakdown of the NHS costs for the East

Table 4.9. Intraregional Distribution of NHS Facilities 1974

Health District	Revenue allocation per head pop. % difference from East Anglia mean		% difference from mean, capital exp. per head, 1948 to 1974
	Hospital	Community services	
Cambridge	+ 19	+ 13.5	+ 83.4
Peterborough	−18.6	−32.6	+ 5.5
Great Yarmouth	−32.9	−12.2	−67.5
King's Lynn	−33.9	−16.5	−39.4
Norwich	+ 12.9	+ 6.1	−12.3
Bury St Edmunds	+ 6.4	− 1.3	+ 11.0
Ipswich	+ 7.2	+ 15.7	−27.2

Source: East Anglian Regional Health Authority, (i) *Revenue Allocation 1975/6;*
 (ii) *Health District Profiles*

Table 4.10. Staffing Levels in East Anglian Health Districts:
 % Differences from East Anglian Mean 1974

Health District	Hospital medical staff per 1,000 total pop.	Hospital nursing staff per 1,000 total pop.	Community nurses per 1,000 total pop.
Cambridge	+ 46.2	+ 6.4	+ 17.9
Peterborough	− 1.9	−21.4	−23.2
Great Yarmouth and Waveney	−19.2	−19.8	− 3.6
King's Lynn	−23.1	−25.3	−26.8
Norwich	− 9.6	+ 13.5	+ 19.6
Bury St Edmunds	− 5.8	+ 11.5	− 8.9
Ipswich	− 7.7	+ 12.3	− 7.1

Source: East Anglian Regional Health Authority, (i) *Revenue Allocation 1975/6;*
 (ii) *Health District Profiles.*

Table 4.11. Intraregional Variation in NHS Service Provision:
% Differences from East Anglian Mean 1974

Health District	% Patients in district treated outside own district	% Patients treated in district but living outside	Waiting list size, acute per 1,000 pop.
Cambridge	12	25	7.7
Peterborough	8	17	9.1
Great Yarmouth and Waveney	23	10	15.6
King's Lynn	21	13	10.8
Norwich	3	20	11.8
Bury St Edmunds	13	27	7.9
Ipswich	2	5	4.7

Source: East Anglian Regional Health Authority, (i) *Revenue Allocation 1975/6;*
(ii) *Health District Profiles.*

Anglia Region by service. It can be seen that the hospitals service takes over 72 per cent of the budget, while the entire school and community services take less than 6 per cent.

Table 4.15 provides similar figures for Norfolk social services and shows the majority of expenditure going to residential forms of care. Administration of the social services is seen to require almost 13 per cent of total expenditure, and the total cost of administration of health services within the East Anglia region, which excludes the central component of administrative costs, is approximately 14 per cent of the total budget for the region. (See Table 2.1.)

Table 4.16 demonstrates that even within the hospital service there are large variations in costs. The costs per in-patient week are greatest for acute hospitals, while comparatively little is spent on patients in long-stay psychiatric and mental handicap hospitals.

Mismatch of Needs and Resources

This mismatch between services and measurable need has now been extensively documented. This has been called the 'inverse care law':

In areas with most sickness and death, general practitioners have more work, larger lists, less hospital support, and inherit more clinically ineffective traditions of consultation than in the healthiest

Table 4.12. Distribution of Social Service Facilities Within Norfolk 1973/4

	All England average	Norfolk	Norwich	Great Yarmouth	Norfolk % diff. from av.
Net expenditure on social services £ per 1,000 pop.	8,433	6,073	11,991	9,664	−28
Fieldwork staff per 1,000 pop.	0.28	0.21	0.47	0.38	−25
Net expenditure £ per 1,000 pop.					
Under 5 years:					
Day nurseries	2,769	162	4,553	—	−94
Pre-school playgroups	189	28	299	—	−35
Under 18 years:					
Net on children	4,740	1,443	5,227	3,665	−69.6
Mentally handicapped	208	307	48	85	+ 47
Age 18-64 years:					
Physically handicapped	182	176	357	173	− 3
Mentally handicapped	251	181	47	—	−28
Mentally ill	74	20	72	—	−72
Sheltered employment	93	55	221	45	−41
Over 65 years:					
Net on elderly	13,121	12,330	17,791	16,669	− 6
Meals	623	330	1,234	581	−47
Sheltered housing	469	615	1,626	91	+ 30
All ages:					
Mother and baby homes	12	2	5	4	−83
Temp. accommodation	77	21	319	18	−72
Domestic help	1,015	833	1,068	1,699	−18
Telephones	31	2	10	26	−93
Aids and adaptations	68	20	92	73	−70
Holidays	38	5	18	15	−87

Source: CIPFA, *Local Health and Social Service Statistics* (1974).

Table 4.13. Revenue Allocation of Addenbrookes Hospital (Cambridge)
and Two Health Districts 1975/6

	£ Revenue allocation
Addenbrookes Hospital (678 beds incl. 178 regional specialty)	6,541,655
King's Lynn Health District (pop. 167,300) all services	3,542,295
Great Yarmouth and Waveney District (pop. 174,950) all services	3,700,331

Source: East Anglian Regional Health Authority, *Revenue Allocation 1975/6.*

Table 4.14. Allocation of Resources for Various Services Within the
East Anglia Region 1975/6

	£ Cost	% of total
Hospital services		
Cambs. AHA	16,011,634	
Norfolk	19,140,866	
Suffolk	14,089,605	
Hospital medical staff paid @ region	2,328,004	
total	51,570,109	72.4
Community and school health services		
School health services	730,270	1.025
Family planning	197,925	0.28
Health education	56,157	0.08
Screening services	1,600	0.002
Health visiting	652,572	0.92
Domiciliary services	1,928,866	2.71
Other	668,044	
total	4,235,434	5.9
Ambulance service	2,066,609	2.9
Regional blood transfusion service	536,926	0.8

Source: East Anglian Regional Health Authority, (i) *Health District Profiles;*
(ii) *Revenue Allocation 1975/6.*

Table 4. 15. Allocation of Resources Within Norfolk Social Services
1975/6

		£ Cost	% of total
Administration		1,388,570	12.8
Field work		1,016,990	9.4
Residential care:			
Homes for elderly		3,927,160	
Other homes		1,684,030	
	total	5,611,190	51.6
Day care:			
Day nurseries		67,800	
Pre-school playgroups		4,500	
Day care for elderly		52,380	
Adult training centres		562,230	
Sheltered workshops		57,110	
Physically handicapped		96,100	
Other		67,680	
	total	907,800	8.4
Community care:			
Domestic help		1,131,570	
Laundry		6,890	
Children in foster homes		146,840	
Family community care		7,190	
Meals in the home		174,940	
Aids and adaptations		50,370	
Telephones		11,650	
Sheltered housing		99,040	
Holidays and recreation		18,240	
Other		79,320	
	total	1,905,340	17.5
Research and development expenses		38,740	0.4

Source: Norfolk County Council, *Report of the County Treasurer 1975/6.*

Table 4.16. Cost per In-Patient Week of Different Services in Different
Types of Hospital as % Cost in Acute Non-Teaching
Hospitals

Type of Service	Long stay	Chronic	Mental illness	Mental handicap
Medical	27	13	26	13
Nursing	65	66	45	40
Domestic	58	60	27	27
Catering	55	48	45	43
Cleaning	68	55	35	32
Total net costs	44	39	32	30

Source: DHSS, *Hospital Costings Returns* (HMSO, London, 1974); P. Townsend,
'Inequality and the Health Service', *Lancet* (1974), vol.1, p.1179.

areas: and hospital doctors shoulder heavier case-loads with less staff
and equipment, more obsolete buildings, and suffer recurrent crises
in the availability of beds and replacement staff. These trends can be
summed up as the inverse care law: that the availability of good
medical care tends to vary inversely with the need of the population
served.[2]

This mismatch has been also shown in the maldistribution of resources
to the community health services: 'there is some evidence that the
greatest propensity of use of community health services is found among
social class V. Where these people are most abundant fewest resources
are available.'[3] A similar picture emerges from study of the psychiatric
services, where 'The same social factors that *increase* the risk of
developing psychiatric disorder greatly *reduce* the chances of reaching
psychiatric services.'[4] In addition, a recent study of the provision of
child health services concluded:

At regional level general practitioners, health visitors and home
nurses are seriously maldistributed — there are fewer of them where
they are most needed. . .Where the standard of living is high the
health of the children is better and at the same time there is more
money to spend in providing hospital beds and other health care
facilities.[5]

Fragmentation of Caring Services

Responsibility for the provision of most caring facilities is at present divided between the NHS and the local authority social service departments. The NHS is administered through the various management tiers which are under the control of the central Department of Health and Social Security. Control over the social service departments is vested in the elected representatives of the local authority and subject only to indirect control from central government.

Patterns of resource allocation are therefore determined in the NHS largely by centralised decision-making machinery, the details being decided at the various management levels. Finance for the service is provided from central funds. The social service budget, after various statutory services have been provided, is determined by the local authority itself, which has to meet at least a proportion of the expenditure from funds raised locally through rates.

There are no clear dividing lines between these two organisations to determine precisely the responsibility for the provision of caring facilities. Acute episodes of physical illness are clearly the responsibility of the NHS, while the supportive care of social workers' fieldwork is the responsibility of the social services. In the middle of this spectrum there remains a considerable grey area where it is not precisely clear who should be providing services and where the best interests of people in need are certainly not served by this division of responsibility. For example, psychiatric patients, while in hospital, are the responsibility of the NHS. Most rehabilitation apparently comes under the scope of the local authority services. This situation can lead to conflict rather than co-operation, as the local authority might prefer people to remain in hospital at the expense of the NHS rather than rehabilitate them at local authority expense. This is naturally expensive in human terms, but also in the total cost to public funds, because institutional care is the more expensive form of treatment.

The lack of co-ordination between the health and personal social service systems has been highlighted by the recent attempts to make the switch of focus away from institutional facilities and to stimulate the development of community facilities. The NHS is attempting to reduce its commitment to institutional care, but the majority of local authorities have not responded with a commensurate build-up of their facilities. This has been fully documented for the run-down of psychiatric hospitals, where the present policy of the NHS, without adequate local authority response in many areas, has led to hardship.[6]

The situation regarding the care of the elderly is exactly similar and, at the same time as the publication of the DHSS *Priorities* consultative document recommending increased provision of local authority domiciliary facilities, a large number of these authorities were announcing further reductions in the standards of services that they were actually providing.[7]

It has been suggested that the necessary conditions for significant co-operation between welfare organisations are that the organisations should have shared goals, that there should be efficient mechanisms for controlling the exchange process and that they should have complementary resources.[8] Our figures show that the resources of the health service and local authority personal social services are not complementary and that there is ample evidence of poor control over co-operation between the services. Furthermore, the present arrangements for joint funding between the NHS and local authority services represent only a very small amount of cash,[9] which is unlikely to be taken up by exactly those authorities where the gap between the services is actually greatest.

In practice the interrelationship between many statutory agencies is much more complex even than between the two major providers of caring facilities. The policies of the agencies providing social security payments, housing facilities, education and educational welfare, etc., all will reflect on the need for and use of the resources of both the NHS and personal social services. In times of economic hardship this interrelationship is demonstrated by reductions in the services mentioned and an increased demand for welfare and supportive services of all types.

The statistics generated by the various caring agencies give no indication of the mismatch between the actual use of the services and the needs of the population served. Service-orientated statistics can only show the use of those services and not the overlap of provision with other agencies or the presence of those in need who fail to reach any of the services altogether. Where community-based surveys have been performed, they have shown tremendous shortfalls and confusion amongst potential recipients caused by the fragmentation of the providing agencies.

The most comprehensive survey available studied the plight of elderly people on discharge from hospital and found that the plethora of services was very confusing for most of the elderly people themselves. The more frail or inarticulate the elderly person was, the less likely he or she was able to understand, apply for or receive the full range of services. It was also strikingly demonstrated in this work that the services themselves were not designed with the needs of the elderly in mind, that they were poorly co-ordinated, and that the services themselves just were not clear about the limits of their own responsibility.[10] Other studies on the co-ordination between the various services for the elderly have arrived at the same conclusion[11] and surveys amongst other client groups frequently demonstrate the dangers of fragmented service provision.[12]

Notes and References

1. J.H. Rickhard, 'Per Capita Expenditure of the English Area Health Authorities', *BMJ* (1976), vol.1, p.299; see also D.R. Jones, 'NHS Resources: scales of variation', *British Journal of Preventive and Social Medicine* (1976), vol.30, no.4, p.244.
2. J.T. Hart, 'The Inverse Care Law', *Lancet* (1971), vol.1, p.405.
3. J. Noyce, 'Regional Variations in the Allocation of Financial Resources to the Community Health Services', *Lancet* (1974), vol.1, p.554.
4. G.W. Brown, 'Social Class and Psychiatric Disturbance', *Sociology,* May 1975.
5. R.R. West, 'Regional Variations in Need for and Provision and Use of Child Health Services in England and Wales', *BMJ* (1976), vol.2, p.843.
6. National Association for Mental Health, *Co-ordination or Chaos?* MIND Report No.13, May 1974.
7. DHSS, *Priorities for Health and Personal Social Services in England* (HMSO, London, 1976); for announced reductions, see Radical Statistics Health Group, *Whose Priorities?*, available from Radical Statistics Health Group, c/o BSSRS, 9 Poland Street, London W1.
8. J. Tibbitt, 'The Social Work/Medicine Interface: A Review of Research', mimeo., Central Research Unit, Social Work Services Group, Scottish Education Department, 1975.
9. DHSS, *Joint Care Planning,* Circular HC (76) 18 (DHSS, 1976).
10. M. Marshall, *The Continuing Care Project* (Age Concern, Liverpool, 1975).
11. L.J. Opit, 'Care of the Elderly Sick at Home: Whose Responsibility is it?' *Lancet* (1976), vol.2, p.1127; T. McKeown, 'Responsibilities of Hospitals and Local Authorities for Elderly Patients', *British Journal of Preventive and Social Medicine* (1969), vol.23, p.34.
12. G.S. Johnson, 'Social Services Support for Multiple Sclerosis Patients in West of Scotland', *Lancet* (1977), vol.1, p.31.

5 CHALLENGES TO THE POWER DYNAMIC

Community Health Councils

During the reorganisation of the NHS administrative structure in 1974 it became politically imperative to include some form of consumer representation. It is now admitted by the architects of the reorganised structure that the community health councils (CHCs) were tacked on to the bottom of the system to provide this function.[1] The central dilemma facing these new bodies is whether they should regard themselves as part of the management structure and attempt to influence planning and the running of the service from within, or whether they should remain at some distance from the administration and attempt change by becoming an advocate on behalf of the community. If the first method is chosen it is possible that the CHCs will be incorporated entirely into the management structure and become indistinguishable from the lay membership of the other health authority levels. More importantly, they may well be identified by the public at large as part of the management of the system and may thereby sacrifice any approachability that they could encourage by remaining separate. It is vitally important that the CHCs should not be seen to be only in the business of concurring with the management or professional groups and then explaining to the community why the establishment acted in the way that it did. This obviously achieves special significance at times when the services are actually being cut. There is no harm in understanding why the management acted in a certain way, but the role of advocate for the community should never be lost from view.

By remaining outside the system, and without any executive power, as at present, the CHCs cannot actually take any decisions and might therefore be considered powerless. The administration can now legitimise any unpopular decisions by claiming that they have been considered by the CHC, while on other occasions dismissing the protests of CHCs because they are not representative of the community at large. The major power groups in the service are already developing methods of varying subtlety to silence or incorporate the disturbance areas created, without fundamentally affecting the power dynamics of the system or altering the way in which decisions about health care are actually made.[2] This central dilemma was built into the system when the CHCs were established during the reorganisation of the service, and it can be seen that the resulting confusion is in the very best interests of the major power groups.

The selection procedures and final composition of the CHCs show great variation throughout the country. Some local authorities have granted all their places on the council to members of the local majority party, others have selected non-councillors to represent them. When voluntary organisations have been selected to provide representatives for the CHC there have been gross anomalies between the different regions, and there are no firm guidelines on how suitable organisations should be selected. The selected members are then unclear whether they have been chosen as individuals or as representatives of their particular organisation. During the selection procedure it is evident that some 'ghost' organisations having few active members are represented, yet they have the same voting rights during selection as the large, well-supported local groups. The resulting confusion leaves the CHCs wide open to criticisms that they are unrepresentative of the community. It is also apparent that the composition of the councils is totally unlike the composition of the communities that they purport to represent. Several surveys have shown that the membership of the councils is predictably more middle-aged and more middle class than the community.[3]

Who then do the CHC members represent? It is apparent that each individual member comes to the council with one or several partisan interests and is unclear how best to develop a balance between competing interests or ideas and how to arrive at solutions that will be for the good of the entire community. It is therefore unlikely that this is the best way to ensure that the voice of the community is actually heard or that a balance between the various competing interest groups is arrived at. There remains considerable opportunity for powerful lobby groups to develop within the CHCs, either on a geographical basis or representing particular diseases or client groups. The problems of the political divisions within the councils has similarly not been resolved. Although most of the members of the CHCs are very easily identifiable politically, e.g., they are often local authority council members, etc., the claim that CHCs should be nonpolitical simply means that in practice the obvious political differences that do exist are never made explicit.

It has been suggested that the functions of the CHCs can be divided into brokerage and activist functions.[4] The 'brokers' see their role as acting as a two-way link between the NHS and the general public, while the 'activists' see their role as keeping the NHS on its toes by examining and criticising the decisions and priorities that the NHS management are taking. Detailed examination of the way that the CHCs have been established and the tools that have been provided for either of these functions certainly suggests that they will be ineffective in both. Either function requires methods of finding out what the community does want, continuous monitoring of the decisions that are being taken by the management and an effective method of communicating with the general public affected by those decisions. Unfortunately it is only too obvious to see that in practice none of these basic tools are available to the majority of CHCs. The budgets of the CHCs are so small that surveying of public opinion becomes impossible and access to the information systems that the councils need for monitoring the management is entirely dependent on the local management of the service whose performance they wish to monitor or criticise. Communication with the general public is often very imperfect, and it is probable that the great majority of ordinary people still have no idea of the existence of the CHCs, the relevance of their activities, or indeed the function that they are attempting to perform.

The debate concerning the structure, composition, statutory power and accountability of the CHCs themselves must continue but should not take up all the energies of the councils themselves or obscure the terrific opportunities that do exist at present to pursue their role as advocate for members of the community. It is probable that only when they can be seen by the community itself to be involved in furthering the interests of that community will they be regarded as relevant by the people they purport to serve. In other words, legitimacy should be conferred on the councils by the community, rather than by attempts to join the statutory bureaucracy in some minor and necessarily impotent fashion.

Even more difficult for the CHCs is the task of concentrating on the *health* of the community rather than on attempts to distribute an illness-orientated service.[5] There is no doubt that ensuring equitable coverage of an understanding and effective curative and institutional service is an important part of the work of CHCs, but this should not detract from the adequate consideration of the *caring* functions of the service. In particular, the CHCs should ensure that services are organised to provide support for informal family and neighbourhood networks.

It may well be claimed that none of this is the role of CHCs as presently constituted. However, there is no reason why CHCs could not act as a powerful focus to discuss these concerns of 'health' in its

widest context. Concentration of effort on the NHS and its
management structure alone will ensure that CHCs follow the consumer
councils within other nationalised industries and become bodies in
limbo, divorced from the real power structure of the NHS and largely
irrelevant to the health of the community.

Challenges from Trade Union Power

Within the structure of the NHS the medical and administrative groups
have retained most of the decision-making power despite the numerical
superiority of the other health service workers. In the past the weakness
of NHS workers was probably due to a combination of factors,
including the wide dispersal of health service facilities in small units,
rather weak union structure and a general acceptance of a subservient,
submissive role with accompanying expectations of low wage levels.
Workers in the health service may well have been attracted to the work
by a commitment to relieve suffering, and this has traditionally denied
them the full range of options used elsewhere in the labour force,
including withdrawal of labour, for fear of the consequences for their
patients.

The increasing power and improved organisational structure of the
health service unions has developed from concentrations of manpower
into larger, centralised units and a growing militancy arising from the
realisation that wage levels in this sector were really very far below
those acceptable in comparable employment outside the NHS.

The introduction (from 1967 to 1974) by the management of various
bonus schemes to control the workers' productivity is seen by some as
a crucial turning point in getting health service ancillary staff to think
collectively about their pay and conditions of work and to establish the
actual machinery whereby those with a common interest met together
to discuss these topics for the first time.[6] The growing numbers of
unionised NHS workers and the increasing firmness of those union's
demands has recently led to improved wages and conditions of work
for ancillary staff and brought them more into line with comparable
employment in industry. In addition, there has been less reluctance to
contemplate the use of the full range of the usual tools of union
activity, including work to rule and the threat of strike action.

It is, however, probably true to say that issues of pay and conditions
of work have provided the major focus for recent union activity within
the health service, and there has been only minor progress in other
legitimate spheres of interest for health service employees of all types.

Entry into Decision-Making

At present health service employees have a very imperfect entry into
the decision-making process of the NHS. It is very striking that each
District Management Team, arguably the most important functional
level of the entire health service, contains three doctors, two
administrators and a nurse, but makes no provision for union members
from the ancillary staff. In addition, none of the new tiers of
management until recently included any representatives of health
service unions. Provision was made in 1974 on Area and Regional Health
Authorities for two members from health service unions,[7] although it
has been ensured that these two members will always be outnumbered
by the representatives of the 'professional' groups on these authorities.

It is possible to view the recent union campaigns against the provision
of pay beds within the NHS in the light of attempts by those working
in the service to countermand the immense power and influence of
those 'professional' groups in whose interest it is to maintain a two-tier
system within the service.[8] During 1974 various health service unions
undertook 'industrial action' to attempt to gain entry into the
decision-making process on the provision of pay beds. These attempts
were at least temporarily successful in opening the debate and
presenting an alternative voice against the powerful consultants'
groups.

The long-term outcome of the campaign against private medicine
within NHS hospitals will be awaited with great interest, but few would
consider that this conflict model for making the views of the majority
of health service workers known to the decision-makers was ideal.

Occupational Health Services for NHS Workers

Despite the evidence of increased risks of disease for many of those
working in the NHS,[9] the failure to provide an adequate occupational
health service to protect the health of workers within the NHS remains
a major anomaly and demonstrates in effect the lack of power the
health service unions at present command. In 1965 the government
appointed the Tunbridge Committee to 'review the existing provision
for the care of the health of hospital staff of all grades'. This
committee commented in its 1968 report:

> For too long the hospital service has failed to give the lead to others
> in the care of staff health that one would expect from an employer
> of well over half a million people and from an organization devoted

to the care of the sick. It is time to start giving that lead.

The TUC has been urging the implementation of this report ever since but ruefully comments in its evidence to the Royal Commission on the Health Service in 1977: 'That lead is still awaited. The health risk factor for staff employed within the service therefore continues unabated.'[10]

The future in this direction looks quite bleak and the 1976 DHSS document *Priorities for Health and Personal Social Services* also shelves the establishment of such a service: 'It is, for example, unlikely that significant expansion in occupational health services [in the NHS] will be possible for the time being.'[11]

Formulation of Long-Term Plans

Because of the unequal distribution of power and the lack of entry into the decision-making and information systems, the trades unions find themselves only able to react to the decisions taken by the major power groups within the NHS. This is especially true in the present atmosphere of reductions in service and the possibilities of redundancy amongst health service workers. In this situation the unions naturally have to fight to protect their members' immediate interests against the closure of various facilities and reductions in staffing levels. However, this reaction can lead the unions into a position of acceptance and defence of the present patterns of health service delivery which at other times they might want to see altered. For example, the trades unions might now struggle to maintain levels of expenditure, employment, etc., in various massive technologically based institutions, although in the present financial atmosphere the maintenance of those facilities might be detracting from the provision of preventive or domiciliary treatment. It can be seen therefore that the unions have a special responsibility to formulate long-term plans for appropriate patterns of caring facilities and then develop their power to ensure that these plans are actually implemented. It is obvious that these long-term plans must be in the interest of both the community and the union membership, and that this will include considerable changes in the actual deployment of labour within the service as a whole.

If what is being advocated is really a switch in priorities and patterns of service away from institutional, high technology and curative practices, then the staffing implications of such a policy must be considered. For example, new types of service delivery may not require lower total levels of staffing, but will certainly require many employees to do different tasks than at present, i.e., community rather than institutional based, preventive *v.* curative, etc. These new skills will require entirely different training and will involve new career structures and remuneration. However, advocating a reduction in certain types of employment within the service has obvious pitfalls for the unions, and this exercise may well be used by the management to cut the services without redeploying staff or building up preventive services.

The shape of the service will therefore remain the same unless the unions can develop sufficient power to ensure that no redundancies are allowed, but that people involved in the changing patterns are retrained in skills that are appropriate to the new patterns of service. It is for this reason that the unions must be encouraged in their fight for a policy of no redundancies and helped in their attempts to establish themselves as a powerful group within the service. However, the immediate aims of the union membership and their struggle to achieve a more powerful status should not detract from much wider, long-term deliberation on the sort of health service that really will serve the best interests of both the community and its employees and exactly what to do with any union power that they might be able to command in the future.

It is possible that developments in the Lucas Aerospace dispute could act as a precedent for action of this sort within the health service. At Lucas Aerospace the unions found themselves fighting to protect their jobs, which they knew to be actually socially destructive, e.g. building weapons of war or making high-technology goods that are ecologically unsound.[12] Their campaign involves the 'right to work and produce socially useful products' and the tactics involve

> working out a complete programme of alternative products which we would make in the event of a cut-back in our traditional products, and we want these products to be socially useful. In order to force the employer to accept this you have got to have a strong organization at the point of production.[13]

It appears that within the health service management and health service unions insufficient deliberation has gone on regarding the staffing implications of any changes in health service delivery pattern. The DHSS *Priorities* document rather weakly states that 'It will also be necessary for some staff to be redeployed, with their agreement, so that the new priorities can be achieved.'[14] However, it gives no indication what this might actually involve in practice. The unions themselves will remain able to react only to others' plans until they develop their own plans for future health service developments, including the implications for their own members, and then develop a strategy for bringing the plans to fruition.

Notes and References

1. R. Klein and J. Lewis, *The Politics of Consumer Representation: A Study of Community Health Councils* (Centre for Studies in Social Policy, London, 1976).
2. T.D. Heller, 'Community Health Councils: The Context for Concern', *Community Health Council News,* February 1977, p.6.
3. Institute for Health Service Studies, *New Bottles, Old Wine?* (Hull University, 1975) and Klein and Lewis, *Politics of Consumer Representation.*
4. R. Klein and J. Lewis, 'NHS Brokers or Activists?', *New Society,* November 1974, p.547.
5. J.B. McKinley, 'A Case for Refocussing Upstream: The Political Economy of Illness', *Behavioral Science Data Review,* June 1974.
6. T. Manson, 'Management, the Professions and the Unions: Power and Ideology in the NHS', mimeo., University of Warwick Sociology Department.
7. DHSS, *Democracy in the National Health Service* (HMSO, London, 1974).
8. N.C.A. Parry, 'Professionalism and Unionism: Aspects of Class Conflict in the NHS', paper presented to British Sociological Association annual conference, Manchester, April 1976.
9. J.N. Harrington, 'Survey of Safety and Health Care in British Medical Laboratories', *BMJ* (1977), vol.1, p.626.
10. Trades Union Congress, *Submission to the Royal Commission on the NHS* (TUC, London, 1977).
11. DHSS, *Priorities for Health and Personal Services in England* (HMSO, London, 1976).
12. Lucas Aerospace Combine Shop Stewards Committee, 'Dole Queue or Useful Projects', *New Scientist,* 3 July 1975, p.10.
13. M. Cooley, *The Right to Work and Produce Socially Useful Products* (Socialist Environment and Resources Association, London, 1975).
14. DHSS, *Priorities,* para.2.1.

6 TOWARDS A COMMUNITY FOCUS

This chapter attempts to explore the possibilities for a re-orientation of the National Health Service towards a 'whole community' approach. It also attempts to discover how far it might be possible to move in this direction using the information and intelligence networks of the caring services as presently organised and suggests reasons why this approach to medical practice does not enjoy universal acceptance.

The Establishment of a 'Community Diagnosis'

At its simplest level, the establishment of a community diagnosis might involve the following components:

(1) Who is ill, and with what disease, in the community?
(2) What might be causing this illness?
(3) What do people do when they are ill?
(4) What facilities and organisations are currently provided for preventing and coping with illness?

Also, might the answers to the first three questions suggest alternative methods of organising these services?

It will be appreciated that this approach does indeed represent a major departure from the traditional ethic of the medical profession and from current methods of planning the caring services. The basic philosophy behind Western medical activity, including the Hippocratic oath, implies that the primary loyalty of the physician is to his patient as an individual.[1] Present-day medical services appear to be organised largely as the sum of these separate commitments.

There are several lines of evidence that would appear to question this traditional individualist focus and support the evolution of an approach to whole community medicine, as represented by the ideas inherent in a 'community diagnosis'.

1. Problems of the Iceberg Phenomenon

Doctors and health services have always been geared to respond to demands from patients when they feel themselves to be ill. It is now evident that this approach only deals with the tip of the iceberg of medical needs and ignores the people in the community with pathological conditions who do not, or who cannot, present themselves for treatment.[2] It includes those who wait until their troubles are so gross that presentation becomes imperative, and treatment is dramatic, expensive and often futile. In addition, there are large numbers of symptom-free conditions that could be diagnosed using presently available techniques but for which diagnosis, in practice, depends largely on chance. It has been estimated from various community surveys that

> for every case of diabetes, rheumatism, or epilepsy known to the GP there appears to be another undiagnosed case. In the case of psychiatric illness, bronchitis, blood pressure, glaucoma and urinary infections there are likely to be another five cases undiscovered. . .[3]

A community survey in Southwark, using simple screening techniques, found that 52 per cent of persons screened needed further investigation and possible treatment.[4]

The knowledge that the bulk of the iceberg exists below the surface presents formidable problems to the medical profession and to the traditions of one-to-one medicine. The debate to determine a way of dealing with the iceberg is causing a cascade of problems.[5]

First of all, should there be attempts to seek out all cases of pathology in the community — the so-called evangelist approach? Would this approach imply that the present state of knowledge can define the limits of normality? In other words, who is ill? The label of 'sick' can, in itself, create problems and even create its own morbidity.

If symptom-free people are diagnosed as having an illness, then this suggests that they should be offered treatment that will positively affect the course of the disease process. This raises all sorts of questions regarding the effectiveness of medical interventions. When examined in a critical light, it appears that many conditions that are presently treated by modern medical methods remain unaffected by the treatment. There have never been controlled trials for many of the regimes that the medical profession now uses routinely.[6]

All these concerns will affect not only the treatment of whole communities, but also the individualistic traditional approach to medicine. Consideration of whole-community medicine has created a challenge to the way in which doctors treat their individual patients, and the introduction of a rational examination of the effectiveness of treatment regimes involves consideration of quality control. If there are some treatments that are of proven effectiveness, how can one stop members of the profession using ineffective treatments that might be expensive or even harmful?[7]

2. The Role of Statutory Services

Before the advent of community-orientated research, it was assumed that the medical profession and the statutory services were of central importance in the diagnosis, treatment and general care of ill people. This rather egocentric orientation has been disturbed by a number of surveys which suggest a different picture.

The Southwark community survey quoted above found that, in the fourteen days before interview, a very small proportion of the people complaining of active disease symptoms had made contact with the statutory medical services, either in general practice or as hospital out-patients. For every medicine prescribed by a doctor, two were being taken on lay initiative, and only 30 per cent of the diagnoses offered had ever been made by a medically qualified practitioner.[8] (See Table 6.1.)

A community survey of women in Camberwell found that 57 per cent of the women who had developed severe anxiety/depression symptoms in the year before the survey had not sought help from the medical services.[9]

Several surveys have established that most of the caring functions for the majority of severely handicapped, chronically sick, and incapacitated elderly who remain in the community are performed by informal networks of relatives, neighbours and friends.[10] The statutory services appear to be of minor importance (see Table 6.2) and are often inappropriately organised to support these informal networks.[11]

Whatever the reasons for the apparent reliance on nonprofessional sources of advice, or the failure of the caring services to actually provide satisfactory levels of care, it can be seen that the picture that might emerge from routine community diagnoses could represent a potent threat to the esteem of the medical profession and lead to changes in the organisation of the present services.

The implications of a reappraisal of the role of the statutory services are enormous. It might be suggested that the services should reorientate themselves to provide meaningful support for the families and friends who do the actual caring. This would not only involve a change in status for the caring professions, but might also involve a commitment for them to share some of their knowledge with the people doing the caring to achieve the maximum benefit. This opens the entire debate about

Table 6.1. Management of the Five Most Common Complaints Found on Survey as Percentage All Complaints in Group

Complaint Group	Visited doctor	Away from work	Bed rest	Asked non-medical advice	Prescribed Medication Medical	Prescribed Medication Non-medical	Diagnosis Medical	Diagnosis Non-medical
Respiratory	4.1	3.0	1.0	0.6	13.0	21.1	37.0	63.0
Tiredness, worry, etc.	3.7	1.7	0.8	0.3	11.1	19.0	19.6	80.4
Rheumatic	5.1	1.6	1.0	0.1	16.4	29.8	39.2	60.8
Digestive	4.2	1.5	1.4	1.4	13.6	36.1	22.7	77.3
Skin	5.0	2.2	1.2	0.8	17.7	50.4	27.3	72.7
Total	4.4	2.0	1.1	0.6	14.4	31.2	29.2	70.8

Source: M.E.J. Wadsworth, *Health and Sickness: The Choice of Treatment* (Tavistock, London, 1971).

Table 6.2.   Home Cases: Visiting of Care Groups

by District Nurse

Care Group	Total	No. being visited	Prop. of total	Average rate Visits/ month	Average duration Mins./ visit	Average intensity Mins./ day
Low	242	56	23.1	5.5	15.9	3.1
Intermediate	58	37	63.8	8.7	24.8	7.7
High	20	19	95.0	11.0	23.9	9.4
All groups	320	112	35.0	8.0	20.4	5.8

by Home Helps

Care Group	Total	No. being visited	Prop. of total	Visits/ month	Hours/ visit	Hours/ day
Low	242	165	68.2	10.1	1.5	0.5
Intermediate	58	34	58.6	13.2	1.5	0.7
High	20	5	25.0	16.0	1.5	0.8
All groups	320	204	63.8	10.8	1.5	0.6

Source: P. Pasker, 'Inter-Relationship of Different Sectors of the Total Health and Social Services System', *Community Medicine,* vol.126 (1971), no.20, pp.272-6.

'professional' sources of knowledge and, therefore, power and authority.

The size of the role of the statutory services is also being critically examined in the historical perspective that is a further part of any full community diagnosis. It appears that the decline in mortality and morbidity levels in Western communities occurred well before the advent of specific medical interventions.[12] Although it remains a possibility that the introduction of certain medical technologies has hastened some aspects of this decline, the exercise would appear to be a salutary lesson to those who imagine that the medical profession and our present services are alone responsible for the enjoyment of our present high levels of health.

This argument has been expanded by a series of authors, both for the Western nations and with regard to certain developing nations. However, much of the work is misrepresented to suggest that modern medical technology has no useful purpose to serve. This is not the case being argued here. But surely the historical perspectives inherent in the diagnoses of whole communities will give a perspective that might diminish the role and importance of technological intervention, and bring into question various aspects of the myopic individualistic focus of much of medicine as currently practised.

Problems of the Distribution of Illness in the Community

The mapping of the distribution of illness in a community will soon establish the great differences in standards of health between the various social classes. Without going through the entire range of evidence, it is possible to suggest that the dissemination of this information will prove uncomfortable to those who suggest that class distinctions are being eroded in contemporary society. It might also be suggested that the medical profession is performing a class role in following their exclusive concern for individual patients at the expense of uncovering the patterns of illness within the entire community.

The evidence shows that, although the mortality rates in all classes are falling, the differential *between* the classes remains the same as ever.[13] This has been shown for standardised mortality ratios and infant mortality rates (see Table 6.3). The separate causes of death applying to men show that 49 out of 85 categories have a higher death rate in social classes IV and V than in classes I and II (see Table 6.4). For women, the figures show that 54 out of the 87 causes of death have a similar class gradient, while only four causes of death show a reversal of the gradient.[14]

These mortality statistics are almost certainly indicators of the morbidity patterns within the community. Unfortunately, only crude estimates of morbidity are available, but these do indeed show a similar disadvantage for the members of the partly skilled and unskilled occupational classes.[15] (See Table 6.5.)

The questions that would be raised by continual and local assessment of patterns of mortality and morbidity might lead to contemplation of the reasons why there are such class differentials in illness. If the reasons are thought to lie in the realms of differences in economic status, nutritional patterns, housing, occupation, etc., this might appear to reduce the role of the medical profession in both the prevention and treatment of the patterns of disease found. More

Table 6.3.   Infant and Neo-Natal Mortality by Social Class

Social Class	Neo-natal mortality		Infant mortality	
	Rate	Standardised mortality ratio	Rate	Standardised mortality ratio
I & II	9.2	79	12.7	73
III	11.8	101	17.2	98
IV & V	13.2	113	20.8	119

Source: B. Preston, 'Statistics of inequality', *Sociological Review,* vol.22 (1974), p.103.

Table 6.4.   Standardised Mortality Ratios of Males Aged 15-64 Years for Selected Causes of Death: England and Wales, 1961 (All Classes = 100)

Cause of Death	Social Class				
	I Professional	II Intermediate	III Skilled	IV Semi-Skilled	V Unskilled
All causes	76	81	100	103	143
Tuberculosis	40	54	96	108	185
Cancer of stomach	49	63	101	114	163
Cancer of lung	53	72	107	104	148
Coronary disease	98	95	106	96	112
Bronchitis	28	50	97	116	194
Ulcer of duodenum	48	75	96	107	173
Accidents (excl. road)	43	56	87	128	193

Source: DHSS, *Prevention and Health: Everybody's Business* (HMSO, London, 1976).

importantly, it might include deliberation on the class nature of society, and what to do about it if it is really causing such excess mortality and morbidity.

4. What Illnesses Are the Community Suffering and How Can They Be Prevented?

Despite popular and medical attention to the diseases that are amenable to advanced technological intervention, it is increasingly evident that these diseases only represent a small fraction of the total illness suffered.

Table 6.5. Numbers of People Reporting Themselves 'Ill' in Each Socio-Economic Group as a Percentage of That Group in England and Wales, 1972

Socio-Economic Group	% reporting limiting long-standing illness	% reporting acute sickness	% reporting limiting long-standing or acute sickness	% of employed reporting absence from work
I	6.5	6.5	9.5	2.1
II	9.0	7.1	14.2	3.9
III	10.4	7.8	16.0	4.8
IV	11.3	7.8	16.6	5.6
V	16.2	9.2	21.9	6.8
VI	20.8	11.3	27.3	9.9

Source: J. Le Grand, 'Distribution of Public Expenditure in the National Health Service', evidence submitted to the Royal Commission on the Health Service, June 1976.

In the more developed countries it is apparent that the 'new epidemics' are chronic degenerative diseases of the cardiovascular system and various malignancies.[16] (See Table 6.6.) Medical intervention has only a minor, usually palliative role in these conditions. It is believed that these diseases are attributable to diet, smoking and general life-style of the population. However, it appears that preventive efforts directed towards these disease entities have been influenced by the individualistic focus of present-day medicine. The DHSS document *Prevention and Health* is subtitled *Everybody's Business,* indicating the general theme behind current thinking: 'To a large extent, it is clear that the weight of responsibility for his own state of health lies on the shoulders of the individual himself.'[17]

This approach to present-day health hazards is also expressed in the Office of Health Economics publication *The Health Care Dilemma,* published in 1975 but having the flavour of previous generations:

If ill health were to be regarded in the same light as social or economic inadequacy this dichotomy (between 'real' and 'social' illness) could be eliminated. Ill health is at present too often incorrectly seen as being unavoidable and a wholly excusable consequence of exposure to external challenge. It should instead

Table 6.6. Mortality Profile of Early Deaths, Canada 1971

Total Deaths	157,300				
Deaths Below Age 70	75,200				
Age Range	0-5	5-35		35-70	
Total Deaths in Age Range	7,600	9,700		58,000	
Major Causes of Death in Age Range	1,600 congenital abnormality	3,300 neo-natal mortality	6,200 accidents	25,700 cardiovascular	3,600 cancer of bronchus and trachea	1,400 bronchitis emphysema

Source: M. Lalonde, *A New Perspective on the Health of Canadians* (Government of Canada, Ottawa, 1974).

perhaps be seen as a failure of mind or body to adapt and cope with the physical, psychological, and social challenges which every human being must experience.[18]

Although the responsibility and potential for each individual to influence his own level of health should not be undervalued, this approach ignores the important perspective that should be part of a community diagnosis. This would include consideration of society's responsibility for preventing illness amongst its members. It would appear unhelpful to encourage people as individuals to stop smoking, overindulging in the 'wrong' foods and leading stressful sedentary lives when there are evidently so many strong influences encouraging, or even ensuring, that people continue to do these harmful things.

Health education with a whole-community perspective would include help for individuals in maintaining their own health, but would also involve consideration of the social factors leading to the creation of ill health. Examples could be taken from all the activities that are now considered legitimate areas for preventive health education. Efforts to stop people smoking as individuals might be expanded to develop an understanding of the influences that create tobacco dependence within society as a whole.[19] This would include scrutiny of the activities of companies promoting tobacco products and the fiscal involvement of the government.[20]

It must remain a source of comfort to the promoters of illness-inducing behaviour that present health education efforts retain their individualist orientation. It is also probable that these various interest groups would resist any change in health education direction that might be required to implement the findings of a meaningful community diagnosis.

Examination of the Patterns of Caring Facilities

The examination of the patterns of caring facilities would be an integral and continuous part of the community diagnosis. Various unofficial attempts have been made to establish patterns of this sort. (See Chapter 4.)

The first picture to emerge would be the age of NHS facilities. Forty-eight per cent of the hospitals in England and Wales were built before 1918, 6.5 per cent before 1850. Of the 2,300 hospitals in Britain, only 41 have been built since 1945.[21]

The geographical distribution is extremely patchy. There are great variations between the regions, but even greater variations at area and district level.

The areas with poor hospital facilities also have poor community services and below-standard preventive facilities.[22]

The areas with the highest proportion of upper social class inhabitants have the highest expenditure on facilities of all sorts.

Acute treatment and all forms of institutional care take the greatest proportion of the budget, while small emphasis is placed on community forms of care or preventive work.

Even within the institutional sector, psychiatric, geriatric and mentally handicapped patients receive much lower standards of care than those with acute conditions apparently amenable to technological intervention.

The change of these patterns over time shows that there has been virtually no progress towards more equitable distribution of services in recent years.

The exposition of these patterns and their static nature raises questions concerning the forces that created these patterns and that ensure the demonstrated inertia. The patterns are evidence that could be used by those who want to alter the patterns of service and press for equity. The reality of the situation will ensure that the members of the groups at present commanding the bulk of resources will resist movement towards equity and resent the production of material that could be used in the movement towards redistribution.

The Present Information System and the Role of the Community Physician

Many of the components necessary for community diagnosis are not available through the routine intelligence networks of the NHS.[23] Most of the examples used here have come from unofficial or semi-official community surveys. In general, the NHS collects information on the state of the service rather than on the illness behaviour or health of the community.[24] There are official statistics relating to mortality levels, the incidence of a few notifiable diseases and various measures of hospital activity, but no statistics regularly collected regarding the state of health of the community or utilisation of primary care facilities.

The material required to establish the patterns of service is all available from official service statistics, but analysis is usually left to independent sources.

Since the reorganisation of the NHS in 1974, 'community physicians' have been employed by the health service. They now take part in management decisions as one member of the six-person District

Management Teams. Prior to reorganisation, most of the people now employed as community physicians were medical officers of health, who were separate from the NHS and who could consider the health of the entire community, rather than simply concern themselves with service considerations.[25]

In addition, the information and analysis that is available to them, as suggested above, primarily concerns the management of the service rather than the health of the community.

Towards a Community Focus

In this chapter we have tried to indicate the components that would lead to the establishment of a community diagnosis and suggest how far the current NHS intelligence networks contribute to building up this picture. It has been shown that making the diagnosis is not a neutral exercise and has implications for the orientation of the medical profession and the organisation of all the services and wider ramifications concerning the nature of society and the processes of change.

The powerful interests maintaining the status quo will tend to resist change that would ensue from the routine production of community-orientated perspectives and might also be antagonistic to the production of any meaningful diagnosis in the first place.

It appears that the intelligence system does not collect relevant non-service data or analyse the data that is at its disposal in such a way that it could contribute to the production of a full community diagnosis. The community physicians who might have been able to generate and collate such information have been incorporated into the management structure during the recent reorganisation, and they will, by necessity, be restricted to management and service considerations.

Notes and References

1. M. Sokolowska, 'Two Basic Types of Medical Orientation', *Social Science and Medicine* (1973), vol.7, p.807; J.G. Freymann, 'Medicine's Great Schism: Prevention vs. Cure: An Historical Interpretation', *Medical Care* (1975), vol.13, no.7, p.525.
2. J.M. Last, 'The Iceberg: Completing the Picture in General Practice', *Lancet* (1963), vol.2, p.28; J. Williamson, 'Old People at Home: Their Unreported Needs', *Lancet* (1964), vol.1, p.1117.
3. M.H. Cooper, *Rationing Health Care* (Croom Helm, London, 1975).
4. M.E.J. Wadsworth, *Health and Sickness: The Choice of Treatment* (Tavistock, London, 1971).

5. W.W. Holland, 'Taking Stock', *Lancet* (1974), vol.2, p.1494; D.L. Sackett, 'Controversy in the Detection of Disease', *Lancet* (1975), vol.2, p.357.
6. A.L. Cochrane, *Effectiveness and Efficiency* (Nuffield Provincial Hospitals Trust, London, 1971); 'Working Papers on Economic Benefits of Restrictions on Clinical Freedom', *BMJ* (1974), vol.2, p.272.
7. *A Question of Quality?* Editor G. McLachlan (Nuffield Provincial Hospitals Trust, London, 1976).
8. Wadsworth, *Health and Sickness*.
9. G.W. Brown, 'Social Class and Psychiatric Disturbance among Women in an Urban Population', *Sociology*, May 1975.
10. P. Pasker, 'Inter-relationship of Different Sectors of the Total Health and Social Services System', *Community Medicine* (1971), vol.126, no.20, pp.272-6.
11. M. Bayley, *Mental Handicap and Community Care* (Routledge and Kegan Paul, London, 1973).
12. J. Powles, 'On the Limitations of Modern Medicine', *Science, Medicine and Man* (1973), vol.1, no.1.
13. P. Townsend, 'Inequality and the Health Service', *Lancet* (1974), vol.1, p.1179.
14. B. Preston, 'Statistics of Inequality', *Sociological Review* (1974), vol.22, p.103.
15. J. LeGrand, 'The Distribution of Public Expenditure on the National Health Service', evidence submitted to the Royal Commission on the Health Service, June 1976.
16. 'Health Trends and Prospects, 1950-2000', *World Health Statistics Report* (1974), vol.27, no.10.
17. DHSS, *Prevention and Health: Everybody's Business* (HMSO, London, 1976).
18. *The Health Care Dilemma* (Office of Health Economics, London, 1975).
19. J. McKinley, 'A Case for Refocussing Upstream: The Political Economy of Illness' *Behavioral Science Data Review*, June 1974.
20. P. Draper, 'Health, Money and the National Health Service', Unit for the Study of Health Policy, Guy's Hospital Medical School, London, 1976.
21. D. Owen, speech to Association of Scientific, Technical and Managerial Staffs conference, 6 December 1975.
22. J. Noyce, 'Regional Variations in the Allocation of Financial Resources to the Community Health Services', *Lancet* (1975), vol.1, p.554.
23. J.N. Morris, 'Tomorrow's Community Physician', *Lancet* (1969), vol.2, p.811.
24. J.A. Muir Gray, 'Specialities within Community Medicine', *BMJ* (1976), vol.1, p.1018.
25. L.M. Mayer-Jones, 'Future of Community Medicine', *BMJ* (1976), vol.2, p.1406.

7 PATTERNS OF MEDICAL PRACTICE IN ENGLAND AND THE THIRD WORLD

The problems of the developed world are usually discussed in isolation from those of the Third World. It is commonly held that our problems are entirely different from those to be found in the developing world and that we can be thankful that we are not in the same desperate situation that can be found 'over there'. Coupled with this belief is something of a criticism of the peoples of the Third World themselves and, in particular, the members of their educated elites, who are thought to be lacking in the devotion which is said to be required to 'get the country out of its troubles'.

These sorts of opinions have led to the development of the aid mentality, where the Western nations are thought to be in a position of strength and can afford to give away some of their surplus, or a portion of their superior knowledge, to help alleviate some of these remote problems. More recently, some radical sociologists and economic theorists have suggested that it has been our intrusion into the affairs of these nations which are now poor that has caused their underdevelopment, and will be a hindrance to their future development. They argue that the more contact an area has had with Western economic and cultural influence, the less real development has taken place there.[1]

Both these theories seem to suggest that the problems of the developing world are indeed different from those of the Western world, and therefore any possible solutions to the problems will rely on separate consideration of two different sets of conditions. The purpose of this chapter is to discuss the possibility that the problems of the Western World and the developing world, and any likely solutions, are identical.

An attempt is made to describe the patterns of health care in the developing nations and the basic similarity of this pattern to that found in England at the present time. In so far as the medical profession can be said to have a dominant professional ideology, it is described, and its effects on the distribution of care shown.

The aid mentality transferred to medicine has led to much of the current thinking about the problems of the health of the people in the Third World. It is thought that 'they' are in a terrible way, undernourished and disease-ridden, and what 'they' want is better coverage of our brand of medicine. In the past, there have been attempts to administer this through large gleaming hospitals, the staff making brief tours into the bush to immunise anyone they could catch and distribute birth control devices to stop 'problems' getting any worse. It has recently become obvious to most people that this effort has been unsuccessful: the people continue to be unhealthy and ever-multiplying.

This insensitive influx of Western medical technology is easy to criticise. It is frequently stated to have been the root cause of the present maldistribution of health care and to have set the present attitudes to be found amongst members of the Third World medical profession. It is now thought enlightened to suggest that what 'they' want is increased emphasis on preventive medicine plus the training of some type of village-level doctors, mainly in public health, providing only a very simple curative service. Even if this approach is the correct one, it is very unlikely that an effective change of this nature will actually take place without a similar alteration in emphasis within our own Western health care delivery system. Rather like the grossly fat parent attempting to stop a child eating between meals, we stand little chance of effecting any change of this nature in other people's affairs until we realise that our own situation is in as urgent need of critical examination. Similarly, while it is easy to criticise those members of the medical profession within developing nations who appear to lack the determination to make the adjustments that we would now consider necessary to achieve this shift of emphasis in health care delivery, we should be fully aware of the attitudes of our own medical profession at home, who are resisting exactly similar changes, and who appear intent only on pursuing their own sectional interests.

The concern here, at this preliminary stage, is not to recommend precise cures for the various ills outlined, but only to suggest that little real progress will be made in improving the health of the bulk of the population in the developing world until we exert similar energy and thought on our own problems, and can be seen to be applying the new standards to ourselves also.

Patterns of Distribution of Health Care

Concentration in Centres of Excellence

It is very well known now that the major part of the health care effort in the Third World is concentrated in the large towns rather than in the rural areas where the majority of the population lives. This has led to the invention of the now accepted phrase 'rule of threequarters' by David Morley, who observed that 'threequarters of the health care effort is concentrated in urban areas.'[2] However, a very patchy distribution is evident in the allocation of health care resources in England. Many of the most needy areas are very poorly supplied with resources, while the metropolitan areas of London and the teaching areas of all the various health regions are well endowed with hospital facilities and staff. (See Tables 7.1 and 7.2.)

In some rural areas, there is a shortage of resources similar to that in rural areas of the Third World. As shown in Chapter 4, the East Anglian region, which is mostly rural, has the poorest provision of health and social services in all England.[3] Total revenue allocation for hospital services is 17 per cent per head below the average for the rest of the country. However, this shortfall is not evenly distributed within the region itself, and, once again, it is the rural districts that have the poorest provision of facilities. Expenditure in the urban teaching district (Cambridge) falls only 13 per cent below the national average, while King's Lynn and Great Yarmouth districts (both very rural) are each more than 51 per cent below average. Capital expenditure per head of population between 1948 and 1974 was over six times greater in the Cambridge district than in Great Yarmouth. (See Table 7.3.) The 1975/6 cost of running a single hospital in Cambridge (Addenbrookes) is almost as much as the entire health services budget for King's Lynn and Great Yarmouth and Waveney health districts. (See Table 7.4.)

Table 7.1. Resource Distribution between Teaching and Non-Teaching Areas: Hospital Expenditure Per Capita 1971/2

Regional Health Authority	% Difference from National Mean	
	Teaching area	Non-teaching areas
Mersey	Liverpool +62	−17.5
South-Western	Avon +14	−24.3
Yorkshire	Leeds + 2	−11.7
West Midlands	Birmingham +10	−29.0

Source: M.J. Buxton, 'Distribution of Hospital Resources', *British Medical Journal* (1975), Supplement 1, pp.345-7.

Table 7.2.   Expenditure on Hospital and Community Health Facilities
in English Regions 1973/4

Health Region	Hospital revenue: % diff. from mean	Community health expenditure: % diff. from mean
Metropolitan London	+ 24.1	+ 5.9
South-Western	− 3.6	+ 4.1
Wessex	−13.6	+ 1.0
Liverpool	+ 7.0	−0.6
Manchester	− 9.1	−1.0
Oxford	−10.1	−1.6
Newcastle	− 8.4	−1.7
Leeds	− 3.8	−4.7
East Anglia	−17.4	−4.8
Birmingham	−14.8	−7.1
Sheffield	−22.5	−7.3

Source: Central Statistical Office, *Abstract of Regional Statistics* (HMSO, London,
1974); J. Noyce, 'Regional Variations in the Allocation of Financial Resources
to the Community Health Services', *Lancet* (1974), vol.1, p.554.

Table 7.3.   Intra-Regional Variations in Health Services Provision:
East Anglia (1973/4)

	Health District		
	Cambridge	Great Yarmouth	King's Lynn
Acute waiting list per 1,000	7.7	15.6	10.8
Hospital revenue: per capita % difference from national mean	−13.4%	−51.2%	−51.9%
Capital expenditure per head: 1948-74	£61.47	£10.90	£20.32
Staff per 1,000 population:			
Medical	0.76	0.42	0.40
Nursing	5.46	3.60	3.83
% patients treated outside district	12%	23%	21%

Source: East Anglian Regional Health Authority, *District Profiles* (1974).

Table 7.4.   Concentration of Resources in 'Centres of Excellence'

	Revenue allocation £
St Thomas's Hospital (London) 1973/4	13,870,000
Average London teaching hospital costs, 1973/4	11,773,300
Addenbrookes Hospital (678 beds incl. 178 regional specialty) 1975/6	6,541,655
King's Lynn Health District (pop. 167,300) all services 1975/6	3,542,295
Great Yarmouth and Waveney District (pop. 174,950) all services 1975/6	3,700,331

Source: East Anglian Health Authority, *Health District Profiles.*

The Emphasis on Curative Medicine

There can no longer be any serious doubt that the present amounts of money allocated to health service budgets in the Third World would be better spent by switching the bulk of provision from the current predominantly curative services towards preventive medicine. This unfortunate situation finds an exact parallel in the distribution of medical resources in Western health care systems. Table 4.14 demonstrates that over 70 per cent of the total health service budget in the East Anglian region is spent on hospital services.

This pattern is a parallel of the national picture: only a very small fraction is devoted to preventive medicine.[4] The detailed examination of the health budget of any region reveals a distribution of resources that would arouse the indignation of the experts in health care delivery if it were to be found in a developing country.

Although it could be claimed that our current level of knowledge is such that there are not many disease states that we actually know how to prevent, this situation will surely continue until we shift emphasis and resources to solving the problems of prevention. The areas in which there is considerable knowledge of effective preventive medicine will serve to illustrate the current maldistribution of resources in this country.

Smoking and Related Diseases. There is now no doubt that cigarette smoking damages lungs, heart, arteries, gastro-intestinal tract, urinary system, and the unborn children of mothers who smoke. Each year,

30,000 people die in Britain from carcinoma of the lung, and over 25,000 from bronchitis.[5] Apart from this human toll, the costs to the economy are staggering. Smokers use the health service more frequently than non-smokers,[6] and over 30 million work-days are lost annually from chronic bronchitis. The anti-smoking campaign run by the Health Education Council had an annual budget of approximately £702,293[7] in the same year that over £70 million was spent by tobacco companies promoting cigarette smoking.[8]

Occupational Health. A crude cost/benefit equation can also be attempted in the field of occupational medicine. Over 741,000 new claims for industrial injury are made each year, and over 17 million days are lost each year following injuries at work, resulting in a bill of over £215 million for the country's industrial benefits.[9] To combat this, the Employment Medical Advisory Service has been established with a budget of approximately £3 million and a staff of about 100 doctors.[10]

The Pursuit of Technological Medicine

Much attention is focused on the undesirability of pursuing advanced technological medicine in the Third World. It appears highly inappropriate that a heart-lung machine is installed, or a complex kidney unit developed, in a country where there is gross malnutrition and where people die for want of simple preventive or curative medicine. Similar distortions can be demonstrated in the 'developed' nations, where the channelling of scarce resources towards the highly complex procedures that can only benefit a few means that the majority are left with a service of very poor quality. The majority of patients in this country are in geriatric, psychiatric, or long-stay hospitals, yet it is exactly these hospitals that remain starved of funds, while no expense is saved aiming at various technological goals. This is illustrated in Table 4.16.[11]

The Medical Profession

Intra-Country Mobility

There is frequent implicit criticism of the members of the medical profession within the Third World. It is said that 'they' won't work in the needy areas and usually tend to migrate towards the large cities where there are already plenty of doctors. They are thought to be attracted to those areas of their countries where they can mix with others of their own social standing and possibly supplement their incomes with private work. Before offering such criticisms, we ought really to examine the distribution patterns of our own doctors within the 'developed' nations.

At its inception, the (British) National Health Service inherited an unequal distribution of doctors and, ever since then, successive governments have attempted to induce general practitioners to work in those areas of Britain most in need of medical manpower. These attempts have been largely unsuccessful, and the doctors tend to ignore the financial rewards in order to practise in more attractive areas, already well endowed with doctors: 'There is everything a doctor needs here, fishing, golf course, walking, not many people', local general practitioner (GP) in Devon; 'My ideal practice would be in a salubrious area with the right middle-class neighbours to consort with. . . stockbrokers, solicitors etc', GP in Essex.[12]

As in the Third World, it is the areas that attract the best-qualified, best-equipped doctors that have the least need of medical care. The areas with the highest proportions of ordinary working-class people attract the fewest doctors. Yet it is these sections of the community that suffer more than their share of the nation's morbidity and mortality. This has led to the description and validation of the 'inverse care law', whereby those most in need of medical care are the least likely to receive it.[13]

The Brain Drain

A proportion of the doctors trained in the Third World leave their country of origin/training to work in those pastures that they consider to be greener. This represents a very sizeable drain of resources for the developing countries and a real boost to the host's medical services. From exactly those countries that are most in need of trained medical personnel, there is a continuous drain of such people. At the end of 1967, Pakistan lost over 2,000 doctors and currently loses over 50 per cent of its annual output straight from medical school. Similarly, Sri Lanka, despite attempted restrictions, loses 120 doctors (50 per cent) of its new graduates each year.[14] Iran loses 25 per cent.[15] Possibly the most amazing story comes from the Phillipines, where the authorities had to hire a football stadium one year to seat all the doctors who had applied to take the qualifying exam to work in the United States.[16]

The benefit of this continuous drain from the Third World falls on our Western health services, which would certainly find it impossible to maintain present standards without the influx of foreign graduates.

In Britain in the mid-1970s, 35 per cent of all hospital doctors were trained overseas, and over 60 per cent of senior housemen were trained in the Third World. They fill the jobs that our own graduates will not take and are diverted towards the unpopular hospitals and the unpopular specialties. Only 19 per cent of teaching hospital doctors come from abroad, while the percentage rises to 39 per cent in all other hospitals.[17]

Before we offer comments about the drain of resources, or even propose possible solutions, we should realise that exactly the same drain continues with our own graduates. Each year, there is a net loss of about 300 doctors, representing the output of more than two medical schools and equivalent to 10 per cent of new medical graduates.[18] It would appear possible that one answer to our own problem, as well as to those apparent in developing countries, might be to attempt to select people for training who are motivated to serve within their own community after qualification, and to make quite sure that the training they receive is fully relevant to the conditions that they will experience in actual practice.

Aspirations

It is probable that the present-day medical profession within the Third World still regards the members of the Western medical profession as the reference group against which they judge their own performance. Thus, the aspirations that are currently found within the Third World have their basis in the West. It might, therefore, be considered unjust to criticise the individual members of the profession within the Third World for wishing to pursue advanced, technological medicine, if this is the dominant aspiration of our own professional groups.

As detailed in Chapter 3, in Britain currently the teaching of community medicine, public health and occupational medicine is minimal and, in some colleges, actually non-existent. In a recent survey of 25 medical schools, 10 had no teaching in occupational medicine at all.[19] Only 4 out of the 12 London teaching hospitals had established departments of community medicine four years after this had been recommended by the Royal Commission on Medical Education.[20] This emphasis is reflected in the career preferences of medical students themselves, and Table 3.3 illustrates that in the three latest surveys, under 2 per cent of students would choose community medicine as their first choice of career.

Once started on their professional life, specialists in public health or community medicine still suffer a very lowly status. They are usually not considered 'proper doctors' by the clinicians, nor are they 'real administrators' according to the professional administrators of the service. There are no specialists in community medicine on the powerful committee that distributes merit awards to consultants,[21] and, although 73 per cent of thoracic surgeons and 70 per cent of cardiologists receive merit awards, only 2.9 per cent of all community physicians are rewarded in this way.[22]

It is frequently noted that the doctors in the Third World all come from privileged backgrounds, and are keen to serve the members of their own social class after qualification. It is thought that this creates a 'cultural gap' between them and the less well-educated and socially inferior patients, especially in disadvantaged or rural areas. There is considerable evidence that such a gap also separates members of Western health care professional groups from the majority of the population they attempt to serve. In Britain, 68.8 per cent of first-year medical students in 1961 were from high social class families, and by 1966 this had risen to 75.7 per cent, although only 18 per cent of the total population were members of these two groups.[23] In the nursing profession in 1972, 52 per cent of those chosen for State Registered Nurse training came from professional or managerial homes, while only 12 per cent came from the families of semi-skilled or unskilled workers.[24]

Thus, it can be seen that our health services are largely run by people who have never experienced anything other than middle-class life and are designed by these people to cater very much for middle-class patterns of illness behaviour. The ordinary people from working-class backgrounds frequently find use of the health care network a confusing and frightening experience. Uptake of services from those sections of the community most in need of care is often very low. This has been demonstrated for the uptake of testing for cervical cancer,[25] family planning services,[26] and the use and acceptance of appointment systems. Similarly, the psychiatric services often present a real obstacle to those who are socially remote from the providers of the service, and who might have a different, less verbal, means of communication from those who can expect to receive the best treatment. This has led to the observation that 'exactly those social factors that *increase* the risk of developing psychiatric disorder, greatly *reduce* the chances of reaching psychiatric services.'[27]

Western Medical Imperialism

It is easy to see that the spread of Western-style medical care throughout the Third World represents a system that has been imposed from without. Western methods of treatment are now accepted by the local 'establishments', often with the attempted exclusion of more traditional methods of treating or accepting disease. The practitioners of traditional medicine may be called quacks (people who pretend to have medical knowledge) by the authorities, but they are certainly still acceptable to people who fall ill, especially in rural areas. The majority are still found to consult traditional healers in preference to, or in addition to, Western-style practitioners, even where these are freely available. Much attention in the Third World is now being directed towards incorporating the acceptability of traditional healers into the design of new health systems. Perhaps we in the West should be prepared to examine our own history, and see if a similar pattern has not occurred in the development of our own services and professional groups.

The predominant method that has developed into the prevailing Western system of treating disease was, historically, only one of several rival ways of dealing with disease. Long before the advent of chemotherapy, and before any really effective medical interventions were being practised, the ancestors of our present doctors had achieved a virtual monopoly in treating disease. Through their close associations with other branches of the establishment, they had succeeded in making most other rival brands of medical treatment unacceptable, even illegal. Thus, before any real skill or success in dealing with pathology had been developed, one particular type of 'medicine man' had become a 'professional', and was already protected by all sorts of registration laws and closed-shop tactics (efforts to exclude newcomers and outsiders). These dominant practitioners were able to claim the much later scientific advances as their very own, and achieve respectability and some measure of efficacy. Their strength in defeating potential opposition was formidable. Possibly the best-documented example is in the history of their professionalisation between the fourteenth and seventeenth centuries, when they actively encouraged and sponsored the witch-hunting of their rival practitioners. The ordinary women of the villages, who were skilled or experienced in dealing with disease, or undertook midwifery, were hounded and denounced as witches for several centuries all over Europe. Their skills were pronounced witchcraft by the newly emergent medical profession and they were tortured and burnt in their thousands.[28]

Both in this country and throughout the Third World, there have always been people who become knowledgeable, experienced and concerned about illness, or who are simply good at caring for others.

The recently dominant Western system, with its rigid, professional barriers, does not realise the potential of these people who are readily available in every village and in most families. Knowledge about illness has become tightly guarded by those professionals whose interest it is to keep tight control over their source of power. Those who would surely be able to care for the sick members of society are denied the opportunity by the prevailing attitudes and actual structure of the health care system. An amalgamation of the technical knowledge, now the exclusive property of a few, with the caring potential within each society would, indeed, be powerful medicine.

Discussion

If the patterns of medical care and medical professional attitudes described here are indeed universal, what are the implications for the promotion of health in the developed world and for assisting the Third World?

(1) First, the aid mentality is surely no longer to be seen as appropriate. Offering portions of our own, very imperfect medical system to the developing nations cannot possibly assist them. Even the 'new improved' packages that enlightened aid-givers now advocate, incorporating community-based projects, etc., stand a reduced chance of success unless we are seen to be taking the same medicine for our own similar condition.

This does not mean that we should stop offering help altogether to the developing world, only that we can no longer offer it from an imagined position of strength. Nor does it mean that we have to wait until we have developed the perfect system of health care delivery to start to export (impose) that new one. Rather, we should accept that many of the problems in the promotion of health are universal and, together with the Third World, we stand some chance of arriving at solutions. Naturally, the exact details are dependent on local social and cultural conditions, but many basic features may well be universal, e.g., prevention before cure, a patient-centred approach, service subject to democratic control, minimal social barriers to receiving treatment.

(2) In the West, we have a certain technical superiority in some aspects of medical treatment and should make this know-how available to the developing world without social or financial cost. However, we must also accept that there are many ways in which we have to learn from the 'developing' countries and their attempts to cope with problems essentially similar to ours.

One of the vital lessons that we should learn is to reject the present separation of health care delivery systems from the other factors that are known to have a direct effect on the health of the population. In some developing nations, an integrated assault is under way on many of the social problems of society, and medicine represents only one very small portion of this programme. Housing, education, income redistribution, agricultural production and nutrition programmes all affect the 'healthiness' of the population more than the actual medical service, and are no longer to be considered separately. Medicine, which is not treated in this country as a political subject, automatically becomes very political indeed. Indeed, if the health of the population is best enhanced by achieving a more equitable distribution of wealth and other of society's assets, then it is through political change that those concerned with the 'healthiness' of their population should be required to act.

Two countries which have received considerable public attention because of great improvement in the health of their populations, China and Cuba, have brought this about through radical alterations in the social and economic distribution of the assets of their societies. Only a very small part of their improved health status can be attributed to changes that have been made in their medical services.[29] This certainly does not mean that we now have to emulate (copy) the health care systems of Cuba or China, only that we should be willing to learn from their experiences and, in particular, that improvements in the measurable health of their people have come about through changes in many spheres, not only the purely medical.

On a much smaller scale, there are many other experiments in developing countries that we should be prepared to learn from. In Guatemala, Carroll Behrhorst is attempting to make social and economic changes on a micro scale. Already these have led to improvements in the health of the people that are his concern.[30] Other experiments are in progress in many of the spheres indicated here as possibly applicable to our own health care system: (1) switching resources to preventive medicine; (2) the use of ancillary workers rather than doctors; (3) multidisciplinary health teams; (4) co-operation with traditional healers; (5) democratic control over the health system. Not all the experiments are successful, but the mistakes are also well worth observing. If indeed the same patterns of maldistribution of resources are present in the developed world as are present in the developing world, then it is very evident that we are lagging well *behind* in our efforts to find viable solution.

(3) Although this chapter has been concerned with the

maldistribution of health care resources and the attitudes and assumptions surrounding the promotion of health in the community, similar problems need examination in every other sphere. Within the global community, some population groups have more than enough of everything, including health care, while others are desperately in need of the necessities of life. However, it is apparently no longer sufficient to divide the world simply into rich nations and poor nations, for within the 'rich' nations there are also a great many who live in poverty. This chapter has attempted to examine whether the same factors that are denying health care to those at the bottom of the social order in rich countries are the same factors denying health care to those at the bottom of the Third World pile. If this is the case, then the only solution to the provision of resources of all sorts to the impoverished members of each society would seem to lie in redistribution of available resources, rather than in adding resources to a fundamentally badly organised system.

The 'trickle-down' theory, whereby the increasing financial rewards that accrue to a country are supposed to trickle down through all sections in order to relieve the plight of those at the bottom of the pyramid, is now under intense attack and certainly is no longer universally accepted. It appears that those at the bottom of the pyramid, waiting, never in fact get the goods, and the gap between rich and poor grows larger. Similarly, if health care resources are added to the system organised in the present patterns, then it is likely that a majority in the developed world, as in the Third World, will still be denied access to what should be regarded as a basic human right.

Notes and References

1. A.G. Frank, 'The Development of Underdevelopment', *Monthly Review* (1966), vol.18, no.4.
2. D. Morley, *Paediatric Priorities in the Developing World* (Butterworths, London, 1973).
3. T.D. Heller, 'The Distribution of Caring Facilities: A Case Study of East Anglia', University of East Anglia Development Discussion Paper No.12 (1976).
4. M.H. Cooper, *Rationing Health Care* (Croom Helm, London, 1975).
5. On smoking, see Editorial, *BMJ* (1973), vol.1, p.503; death figures are in DHSS, *On the State of the Public Health* (HMSO, London, 1973).
6. J.R. Ashford, *British Journal of Preventive and Social Medicine* (1973), vol.27, p.8.
7. Health Education Council, *Annual Report, 1973-4*.

8. 'Talking Politics', *Lancet* (1975), vol.1, p.912.

9. DHSS, *Annual Report* (HMSO, London, 1974).

10. Employment Medical Advisory Service, *Annual Report 1973-4* (1974).

11. P. Townsend, 'Inequality and the Health Service', *Lancet* (1974), vol.1, p.1179.

12. J.R. Butler, *Family Doctors and Public Policy* (Routledge and Kegan Paul, London, 1973).

13. J.T. Hart, 'The Inverse Care Law', *Lancet* (1971), vol.1, p.405.

14. B. Senewratne, 'Emigration of Doctors', *BMJ* (1975), vol.1, pp.618, 669.

15. H.A. Ronaghy, 'Physician Migration to the USA', *Journal of the American Medical Association* (1974), vol.227, no.5, p.538.

16. Editorial, 'How Many Doctors?', *Lancet* (1973), vol.2, p.1367.

17. *Doctors from Overseas* (Community Relations Commission, London, 1976).

18. Editorial, *Guardian,* 8 October 1975; *see also* House of Commons. Written Answer, 18 March 1976.

19. H.A. Waldron, 'Undergraduate Training in Occupational Medicine', *Lancet* (1974), vol.2, p.277.

20. 'Who's for Community Medicine?', *Lancet* (1972), vol.2, p.1297.

21. S. Brown, 'Examination of the Distinction-Award System', *BMJ* (1975), Supplement 1, pp.162-5.

22. DHSS, *Annual Report 1974.*

23. *Report of Royal Commission on Medical Education* (HMSO, London, 1968).

24. *Report of the Committee on Nursing,* Cmnd.5115 (HMSO, London, 1972).

25. K.J. Randall, *Lancet* (1974), vol.2, p.1303.

26. M. Bone, *Family Planning Services in England and Wales* (HMSO, London, 1973).

27. G. Brown, 'Social Class and Psychiatric Disturbance', *Sociology,* May 1975.

28. B. Ehrenreich, *Witches, Midwives and Nurses* (Compendium Press, London, 1974).

29. S. Rifkin, 'Health Strategy and Development Planning: Some Lessons from the People's Republic of China', *Journal of Development Studies* (1973), vol.9, no.2, p.213; V. Navarro, 'Health, Health Services and Health Planning in Cuba', *International Journal of Health Services* (1972), vol.2, no.3, p.397.

30. C. Behrhorst, 'The Chimaltenango Development Project in Guatemala' in *Health by the People* (World Health Organization, Geneva, 1975), chap.12.

8 ADMINISTRATIVE FUTURES

The distortions outlined in Chapter 4 are apparent to the administration and those at the political head of the service.[1] In 1976 two major policy documents attempted to find ways of overcoming some of the major disparities in the service and to make readjustments both between the various sectors of the service and between the geographical regions.

The consultative document *Priorities for Health and Personal Social Services in England* was published to present DHSS opinion regarding the switch of some resources away from acute, curative, hospital-based, high-technology medicine and towards building up the community services for the elderly, mentally ill, mentally handicapped, and long-stay patients.[2] Chapter 2 has demonstrated that this switch of priorities *cannot* take place given the present power structure within the health service. The switch will be resisted by those powerful factions that have already distorted the system into its present shape. The consultative document makes no mention of these problems of implementation, and further examination in some detail of the precise priorities that have been suggested indicates that the DHSS actually does not envisage any real change in the shape of the caring services in the future.

In general the priorities can be summarised as a switch away from general acute hospital and maternity services, an increasing emphasis being placed on prevention, primary and domiciliary care, services for the mentally ill and handicapped and the elderly.

However, detailed examination might suggest that in fact the proposed change in emphasis will leave the service very much in the same shape as at present, and, more importantly, will have little effect on the people who are presently in receipt of the poorest services.

The Emphasis on Primary Care

The figures in the consultative document project that there will be an average 3.5 per cent growth rate in primary care services between 1975/6 and 1979/80. However, this figure looks considerably less impressive when pharmaceutical services are not included in the total.[3] (The reasons why the cost of the pharmaceutical service is rising so fast are discussed in Chapter 2.)

Table 8.1.   Current and Capital Expenditure

	1975/6 £m	1979/80 £m	% average growth per annum
Primary care sub-total	742	851	3.5
Primary care minus cost of pharmaceuticals	430	469	2.2

Source: DHSS, *Priorities for Health and Personal Social Services in England* (HMSO, London, 1976).

Furthermore, the rapid growth in numbers of the elderly, who are known to be heavy users of the primary care services, and the increased capitation fees that are paid to general practitioners looking after elderly people, will absorb a considerable proportion of the annual growth rate remaining.

Thus, although it is easy to predict that the service will be more costly in the future, this unfortunately does not necessarily ensure that the standards of care for people using the service will be greatly improved.

The priority given to primary care within the entire health service can also be seen in the document. Current and capital expenditure together is projected to increase from 17.6 per cent to only 18.4 per cent of the total from 1970/1 to 1979/80, while the current expenditure alone is projected to *fall* slightly, from 19.3 per cent to 19.2 per cent. Health centre capital expenditure is also projected to fall from £23 million in 1975/6 to £17 million in 1979/80.[4]

Preventive Efforts

Despite the rhetoric in *Priorities for Health* and in the DHSS discussion paper *Prevention and Health*,[5] data in *Priorities for Health* show that the proportion spent on prevention is very small, and retains the same priority over the period projected.[6] In particular, the problems of occupational health appear to be ignored, although *Prevention and Health* states: 'If the whole of the male working population had had a sickness absence rate equivalent to that reported by professional classes there would be an annual saving of about 100 million working days.'[7]

In addition to this, over 800,000 claims for industrial injury benefits are made each year,[8] and almost 250,000 pensions are paid annually to those with industrial injuries or to their widows.

The Employment Medical Advisory Service remains a small, poorly funded organisation under the care of the Department of Employment rather than the NHS. Occupational health services *within* the NHS itself will not be expanded (*Priorities for Health,* para.2.10), and this might be seen to indicate the priority afforded to this vital aspect of preventive medicine.

Although *Priorities for Health* accepts that preventive efforts and health education should become part of the general work of all sections of the caring services, and in particular of the primary care service (para.3.24), the section on preventive health (paras. 3.23 to 3.26) might easily be criticised as pure rhetoric in the absence of any real diversion of funds to this sector.

Services for the Mentally Ill

Table 2.6 shows that there has been no recent proportionate increased spending on providing services for the mentally ill. However, hope is again created in *Priorities for Health* (para.8.10): 'We regard the development of services for the mentally ill as a major priority.' However, analysis of Figs. I and II (pp.6-7) in *Priorities for Health* shows that the priority is still not reflected in the future projected financial distribution between the sectors of the service. Current and capital expenditure on services for the mentally ill as a percentage of the total is projected to be 8.2 per cent by 1979/80, which is the same percentage as in 1970/1, while current expenditure alone is projected to *fall* over the same period from 8.5 per cent (1970/1) to 8.0 per cent (1979/80).

Table 8.2.   Services for the Mentally Ill

	% of total expenditure		
	outturn 1970/1	provisional 1975/6	projected 1979/80
Current and capital	8.2	7.8	8.2
Current	8.5	8.0	8.0

Source: DHSS, *Priorities for Health and Personal Social Services in England* (HMSO, London, 1976), pp.6-7.

The Gap To Be Filled. . .(and the problems of joint funding)

The figures in the consultative document give some idea of the gap between present provision of services and the 'National Requirement Guidelines'. (See Table 8.3.)

It can be seen that in many cases there is a considerable gap between the current level of services and the levels that are considered satisfactory. The proposed 'growth' in these services will therefore in the first instance be required to bring the services up to a reasonable standard, and should not necessarily be presented as a real switch of resources to the various services to give them a positive priority.

The consultative document suggests that it will take 25 years for the services for those suffering from mental illness to achieve the White Paper guidelines.[9]

It can be estimated that services for the elderly will similarly take a great many years before acceptable standards of service are achieved. Table 8.4 estimates the number of years required for some services for the elderly to achieve the standards proposed as national guidelines. The picture presented of the gap between actual provision and the required standards is complicated by the local variations in standards. There are enormous variations in the present levels of provision, and even the proposed rates of growth would mean that the people in many areas would have to wait much longer than the average figures estimated in Table 8.4 before satisfactory services become available. It is also probable that exactly those authorities with the poorest current services are the least likely even to maintain the target growth rates suggested in the consultative document.

For example, Table 8.5 shows that in Norfolk, the provision of almost all services is well below the national average. In addition, there is a very rapidly growing population of elderly people in the country. The County Council Social Services Committee, however, is cutting back exactly those services that were singled out in the consultative document to receive priority. It is quite evident that, given these conditions, and following the present policies, talk of priority for these services is pure rhetoric, and the guidelines suggested will never be met in the County of Norfolk.

In addition, there are tremendous demographic variations throughout the country (see Table 8.6). Those authorities which have a favourable demographic pattern might be able to maintain a growth rate as suggested, while those with a rapidly rising population of elderly people may find themselves unable to do this.

Table 8.3. Summary of Current Percentage Shortfall

	1974 level of service	National requirement guidelines	Shortfall as % of requirement
Services for mental illness			
Local authority day care	5,000	30,000	−83
Residential places	4,000	12,000	−66
Services for the elderly			
Home helps per 1,000	6	12	−50
Meals served weekly	600,000	1,300,000	−54
Day centre places per 1,000	2	3-4	−50
Local authority residential facilities	18.5	25	−26
Geriatric hospital beds	8.57	10	−14
Services for the mentally handicapped	(proposed by 1985)		
Residential care	9,500	22,000	−57
Training centres	32,000	60,000	−47

Source: DHSS, *Priorities for Health and Personal Social Services,* (HMSO, London, 1976).

Table 8.4. Services for the Elderly

	Growth per annum %	Current shortfall as % of requirement	Years to achieve target
Home helps	2	50	35
Meals on wheels	2	54	37
Day centres (+600 pa)	5	50	16
Local authority residential care (+ 2,000 pa)	2	26	15

Source: C.J.H. Williams, 'Could the Consultative Document Have Its Priorities Wrong?', *BMJ*, vol.2 (1976), p.956.

Table 8.5.   A Profile of Norfolk Social Service Provisions 1976/7

	Ratio per 1,000 pop.	DHSS Guideline	Shortfall as %
*The Elderly (ratio per 1,000 over 65 years)			
Residential care	17.1	25	−31.6
Day care	1.2	3-4	−64.5
Home helps	4.65	12	−61.2
Meals on wheels	79.0	200	−60.5
The Physically Handicapped			
Residential care	3.6	30	−88
Day care	19.5	30	−34.9
The Mentally Handicapped			
Residential care	14.3	60	−76.2
Day care (adult training centres)	90.4	150	−39.7
Children — Residential Care			
	30 places provided by local authority		−55
The Mentally III			
Residential accommodation	no places provided	4-6	−100
Longstay accommodation	3.9	15-24	−90.1
Day centres	3.8	60	−93.6

Source: Data from Norfolk County Council, Social Services Committee 1976.
(*the ratio are per 1,000 total pop. except for the elderly)

There is a varying response by local authorities to the current financial situation and, while many chose that social services should continue to grow relative to the other services under local authority control, this is by no means a universal decision, as Table 8.7 shows.

The Problems of Joint Funding

Throughout the consultative document, there is considerable emphasis placed on the hope that much of the gap will be filled by use of the joint funding arrangements as described in DHSS Circular HC (76) 18.

Table 8.6.   National Demographic Variations

Region	Population aged 65 years and over (thousands)		
	1976	1981	% growth 1976-81
England	6,535	6,856	+5
Yorkshire	501	515	+3
East Anglia	268	286	+7
NW Thames	455	488	+8
NE Thames	519	538	+4
SE Thames	588	593	+1
Wessex	422	459	+9
Oxford	266	289	+9
North Western	580	593	+3

Source: DHSS, *Health and Personal Social Services Statistics 1975* (HMSO, London, 1976).

Table 8.7.   Social Services Growth Rate

	% of 116 authorities surveyed
Over 5% growth	20%
Up to 5% growth	44%
Nil growth	24%
Cuts in real expenditure	12%

Source: British Association of Social Workers Survey, Birmingham, December 1975. Available from BASW, 16 Kent Street, Birmingham.

However, the actual amounts set aside for this scheme presumably come from the total NHS budget in any case and are quite small amounts of money. By 1980 only 0.58 per cent of the total budget will be available for this purpose. For the reasons suggested earlier, we can anticipate that the options to use this method of funding will only be taken up by relatively progressive authorities where the shortfall in services is not the most severe.

Priorities – Rhetoric?

The proposals put forward do not really represent a shift of emphasis or any real change in priorities. There appears to be great variance between some of the stated priorities and firm commitment of financial resources. The financial implications of the forthcoming demographic changes (most particularly the rapid rise in the numbers of the elderly) will affect different sectors of the service in varying proportions. Because of this, the proposed 'growth' in some sectors will be entirely absorbed simply in maintaining services at the present level to cater for the increased numbers of elderly people. The gap between some of the services that are currently provided and the level of services to be considered of reasonable standard is very large indeed. This gap varies throughout the country. Much of the 'growth' that is planned in the various sectors is needed simply to attempt to bring substandard services up to an acceptable level, and can hardly be considered to represent a meaningful shift of emphasis in the services selected for this treatment.

Where the gap is, in fact, being closed, it will be a great many years before satisfactory standards are reached and, in some local cases, it can be shown that the gap is indeed becoming wider.

The Realities of Resource Allocation

The second major government report, *Sharing Resources for Health in England,*[10] is an attempt to start the movement towards geographical equity between the fourteen English regional health authorities. For the first time, an attempt has been made to assess the needs in the various regions, and then allocate resources accordingly. This is obviously an improvement over the previously almost random allocation of resources, which seemed to rely mainly on historical chance. There are serious methodological criticisms concerning the Resource Allocation Working Party (RAWP) report. The most serious is the use of mortality statistics as an indication of morbidity, and thus as an indication of need. It is possible that need for caring facilities, however, is greatest in areas of low mortality simply because people live longer and will require increased amounts of care in their old age. In addition, the distribution of resources below regional level is imperfectly dealt with in the report.[11] Each region is able to decide on resource allocation to its various areas and districts. It is still possible that disparities at district level, where the services are actually provided, will become even greater. This was the case in 1975/6 in the East Anglian region when the previous resource allocation formula provided additional 'development' funds for the region. In fact the richest area per head of population (Cambridgeshire) also received the largest slice of the development money. Within the areas the distribution was again unequal; for instance, in the Norfolk area the Norwich Health District, with a revenue expenditure per head of population on hospital and community services 40 per cent greater than the Great Yarmouth District, also had a larger allocation per head of the additional funds.

It is also evident that in those 'rich' regions where such additional money is not available and cuts in the services are being made, the cuts are made without reference to 'needs' in such a way that the impoverished parts of the region are left even more deprived than previously.[12]

The entire report is open to the same criticisms levelled at the *Priorities* document, in that it does not face up to the problems of power in the service or the feasibility of their recommendations actually being implemented. There is already growing evidence that the power structure within the service will prevent the effective implementation of the report. Already the findings are being vigorously fought by those sectional interests that feel themselves to be hard done by the suggested formula.[13] Those geographical regions, especially those in metropolitan London, have received more money in the past precisely because of their power, and will now use this power to resist the effects of re-allocation of resources. Similarly, the medical profession will fight to maintain the status quo.[14] In the East Anglian region the largest single item of the additional 'development' funds for use at regional level went to pay the increased merit awards for the top consultants. The largest expenditure of these new funds at area level went to pay for the costs of the new Junior Hospital Doctors' Contract. In the Cambridgeshire area increased salaries of junior doctors has taken up more than 50 per cent of the total development money, which was surely intended to improve services for the patients.[15]

Apart from the various sectional and methodological criticisms, the entire concept of resource allocation is being vehemently opposed by some powerful sections within the medical profession. A letter in *The Times* from a professor of surgery at a leading London teaching hospital in 1976 said:

At first sight the transfer of finance, equipment and manpower from the better developed to the poorer areas is plausible and seems fair. Unfortunately medical progress and excellence do not work like this. Advances are not made on a wide, evenly distributed basis.

They tend to be made in the leading centres and after a period to be adopted generally.

We have only to look at medicine in the world as a whole to see where it [resource allocation] leads. To the East we see several countries which have adopted this policy of devolution and dispersal of resources. The chief of them has produced no notable advance in surgery since the War. To the West we see America where excellence is encouraged. This year workers in American centres won all of the Nobel prizes for medicine.

Do we also, like the East want to decline into mediocrity? Do we wish to have to tell our patients affected by serious or complicated illness that they will achieve better advice and help across the Atlantic? These things will happen unless the 're-allocation' policy is reversed.[16]

The hospital in which the author of this letter works itself consumes over £29 million of the NHS budget each year. This is equivalent to the *total* expenditure on all the hospitals, community health services, etc., in the health districts of Bury, Peterborough, Ipswich, King's Lynn, and Great Yarmouth, serving well over 1 million people.

The RAWP document gives a clear indication of the management ideology of the service which is concerned to produce a statistical equity of services, but appears unconcerned with the problems of the appropriateness of the services provided or considerations of the quality. Although the stated objective, which is to provide 'equal access to health care for people at risk', is laudable, the type of reallocation of resources envisaged in the report is only one aspect of a wider problem. There is increasing evidence, for instance, that access in geographical or financial terms is only one part of the problem of differential uptake of services that would otherwise appear to be theoretically without access problems. In other words, where access is apparently no problem, i.e., the service is near at hand and free at the time of use, enormous differences remain such that those who, it is believed, would receive most benefit from use of the services are actually the least likely to take them up.[17] This problem is clearly a problem of certain characteristics of the service provided and of its quality and perceived relevance to the people for whom it is intended. It is evident that this is not being dealt with by the current management and professional concerns, intent on geographically equal 'delivery' of a service without adequate reference to the properties of the service that is being offered.

Summary

The failure of both of the major documents of 1976 to deal with the realities of power distribution and problems of implementation, their failure to grapple with real shifts in service emphasis and problems of the quality or appropriateness of the 'delivered product' indicates that the futures envisaged by the administration are similar to the present structure, function and performance of the system. The gross distortions within the NHS will remain, and power will continue to be distributed in such a way that the best interests of the total community do not appear to be served.

Notes and References

1. D. Owen, *In Sickness and Health: The politics of medicine* (Quartet Books, London, 1976).
2. DHSS, *Priorities for Health and Personal Social Services in England* (HMSO, London, 1976).
3. DHSS, *Priorities for Health*, Annex 2, Table 1.
4. Ibid., Figs. 1 and 2.
5. DHSS, *Prevention and Health: Everybody's Business* (HMSO, London, 1976).
6. DHSS, *Priorities for Health*, Annex 2, Tables 1 and 2.
7. DHSS, *Prevention and Health*, p.53.
8. DHSS, *Annual Report 1974*, Cmnd. 6150 (HMSO, London, 1975).
9. DHSS, *Priorities*, para. 8.12. See also T.D. Heller, 'Dismantling the Welfare State', *Poverty*, December 1976 (Child Poverty Action Group, London).
10. *Sharing Resources for Health in England*, Report of the Resource Allocation Working Party (HMSO, London, 1976).
11. T.D. Heller, *Guardian*, 4 October 1976.
12. G. Dain, *Guardian*, 30 November 1976.
13. 'Compelling Needs of our Hospitals', *BMJ* (1976), vol.2, p.864.
14. 'The End of Excellence', *BMJ* (1976), vol.2.
15. Heller, *Guardian*, 4 October 1976.
16. J.B. Kinmouth, *The Times*, 30 November 1976.
17. J.B. McKinlay, 'Some Approaches and Problems in the Use of Services: An Overview', *Journal of Health and Social Behaviour* (1972), no.13, p.115.

9   DESIGNING THE FUTURE HEALTH SERVICE

This exploration is not a concrete design or plan for the structure of the health service of the future, but rather a series of building blocks which are necessary components for the development of a healthy society.

One of the building blocks is the development of a concept of health that is entirely different to that currently held. We must move away from considering health as something that can either be delivered by doctors, or is the resultant after all bodily disease has been eliminated. In the same way that it would appear inappropriate to develop a new health system and then introduce it to (impose it on) the community, the novel philosophy of 'health' should be the result of a continuing exploration within the whole of society. This exploration should be the aim of any service that concerns itself with health, however vague and tenuous this might appear at present.

It would appear impossible to separate the health components of any society from almost any other area of social action or social policy. Even using current concepts of health, there is no area of activity that cannot be shown to have an effect on the health of the people. Yet the health services remain in a separate compartment for use when people become ill. Our design must therefore be envisaged as one part of a design for all social policy, continuously evolving to meet the needs of the people.

This greater social policy, and its health component, should become one part of change and should not be used to prevent change. If there are certain functions of society that are creating the need for some sort of social intervention, then the policy should not only involve the repair of the casualties, but should also attempt the changes needed to avoid them. Where change is necessary, it should become part of social policy, e.g., if the shape of society is inimical to the health of its people, then the health service should be concerned with changing the shape of society, not simply with patching up more and more of its casualties.

These social policies must become central to society, not — as at present — conceived as appendages which society can afford when economic times are good. Social policy of this nature *is* society and cannot be neglected in times of economic gloom or be used as an economic regulator to lead us into times of boom.

The present shape and distortions of the NHS and other areas of

106

social intervention are mirrors of the shape and distortions present elsewhere within society. Those who seek to iron out the distortions in both are divided between those who suggest that the NHS will change only after society has undergone transformation, and those who feel that the way to change society is through changes in structures such as the NHS. It remains, however, the hope of the policies envisaged in this 'design' that they might serve both to illuminate, and act as a catalyst for, policy changes in other sectors of society.

A Spectrum of Care

Whatever the shape of society, or of the preventive health services, a certain number of people will always come to be in need of caring facilities. The present artificial divisions between the numerous caring agencies leads to confusion and low uptake of services. Our design anticipates the development of an appropriate spectrum of care wherein all caring facilities are part of a co-ordinated whole. An example might be taken from the care of the elderly; the spectrum would include the facilities for technological medical intervention, provision of less intensive institutional care, domiciliary support services, income maintenance schemes, local community activity, housing and transport assistance, and family and self care. A similar spectrum of care could be envisaged for the members of other groups in need.

The resources side of the equation needed to provide such a spectrum requires the development of a theory of community resources which includes all the resources available to that community, not simply the financial and technical/professional. The accounting system should include family and informal networks of caring and should develop the concept of patients as resources rather than passive consumers.

The balance between central government and local control of these activities is of crucial importance. The entire spectrum must be responsive to local needs and aspirations, yet it is possible that central government guidelines and experience could also be valuable. It is envisaged that the bulk of funding for these activities will come from central funds, but that the priorities and shape of the local service will be decided through a local decision-making apparatus. In this way it should be possible to avoid the further development of an increasingly massive central bureaucratic machinery disallowing the active entry of local democratic participation and accountability. An emphasis on local decision-making might create a range of services that is even more uneven than at present, but central government control over the total quantity of financial resources would lead to a more equitable financial distribution.

Within the various components of the spectrum of care, the design envisages a review of the decision-making power. All the contributors to the spectrum should share in decision-making, certainly including the recipients of care. The supremacy of the medical profession should be replaced by an approach that will include all the members of the extended team, the consumers of care and their families. At the level of professional/consumer interaction, it is similarly envisaged that decisions will be arrived at through joint involvement rather than by reliance on professional dominance.

Implicit Functions

No Responsibility without Power

At each level of the system there will be a revision of responsibility. Thus the regions become responsible for the people in their region, the entire team becomes responsible for the care spectrum in their community, and people themselves become responsible for their own health. This can only work if power is also distributed in this fashion and the regions, teams, and people themselves have the power to bring about actual change. Thus patients' committees, community health councils, local health authorities, etc., should not be asked to take decisions without being given commensurate power of control over those factors that do affect them. For instance, there is no point in establishing a patients' committee for a group practice of GPs if nothing happens when they take decisions. (This scheme represents a redistribution of power away from the present majority-holders — the administration and the medical profession — and resistance to these measures might therefore be expected.)

Education and Change

The primary function at each level becomes one of education. This should never be envisaged as a one-way process in which holders of knowledge (power) impart selected portions of it to those on the next rung down the ladder. If a real education process continues at every opportunity and in both directions, and in every sector of the design, then those with responsibility and power will gain the knowledge to develop a system that more accurately reflects the needs of the people within the society. This should include the development of the new philosophy of health discussed at the beginning of this chapter. For example, the present holders of power within the health service administration legitimise this power by claiming that the public do not understand much about health service matters: 'If you asked them, they would want a large hospital in every small town.' The new design relies on the expectation that as the power/responsibility/education process developed, 'they' would decide on the fundamental importance of preventive measures, the use of appropriate technology, etc., etc.

Similarly at professional/consumer level, the supremacy and decision-making monopoly of the profession relies on the unequal levels of knowledge of the two segments, who should surely be partners in decision-making. (It seems unlikely that the present holders of knowledge will always give up this source of power lightly.)

A Possible Shape

Although it is not the function of this first exploration to lay down a rigid plan for the health services of the future, it is possible to suggest a shape that the services might develop, using the general principles outlined in the preceding sections.

The basic unit would appear to become a primary care team, controlled by the community that it serves. The composition of the team and its caring functions would be of much wider scope than in established primary care teams, and would include general medical practitioners, social and community workers, those concerned with legal and welfare rights and those concerned with income maintenance. The primary care team would have a number of resources at its disposal, including access to technological medical facilities, institutional, community and domiciliary support facilities and close linkages with informal networks providing caring facilities.

The informal networks and family and self care would be encouraged to develop and replace the professional facilities wherever possible. This might come about through the education/ power shift described above and through access to 'professional' resources of facilities and finance.

In addition to the function of crisis intervention at times of medical and social stress, the foremost explicit function of the team would be activity leading to the prevention of such crises. This involves all the standard public health and health education efforts but, in addition, would include functioning to change those factors that are inimical to the health of the community. This does not exclude activity in the overtly political areas of environmental, occupational and all 'social health' matters.

10 RESTRUCTURING THE HEALTH SERVICE

Although we have dealt with a wealth of statistics in the preceding sections, we have attempted to present them from the perspective of the people for whom the services are intended. We could conclude by listing again the *effects* of the present shape of the services on the community at large:

(1) In many geographical areas there is a real deficiency in the standards and availability of quite ordinary services of all types.

(2) People suffering from certain sorts of illness receive a standard of services that is much lower than the ideal, and generally lower than that enjoyed by those suffering from other, usually acute, illnesses.

(3) The caring services as a whole are fragmented to the extent that it is difficult for those in need of such services to understand, or to apply for, the range of services that might be of benefit.

(4) The health and caring services as presently organised have only a minor, possibly diminishing, role in caring for people when they are sick.

(5) Decisions on services are taken far away from those who are affected by the decisions. This applies to individuals when they are sick, or when they are trying to remain healthy, and also to whole communities when considerations of service development are made. Similarly, those working in the service are remote from the decision-making process.

(6) Preventive services are underfinanced, under-researched, and underdeveloped compared with the services concerned with the treatment of illness that might possibly have been prevented in the first place.

(7) The current shape of the health service has become the norm for much of the rest of the world. In the developing countries the effects of the adoption of this type of service are particularly devastating.

(8) Wherever in the world health services of this shape have been introduced, there is no good evidence that they are *effective* in reducing the levels of disease in that country.

It has been the purpose of this study to show that in some part these distortions and adverse effects have been caused by the relationships

110

of power within the NHS, and that these relationships will also tend
to work against ironing out these distortions in the future.

It has been shown in detail that in the present financial climate no
real changes are actually anticipated by the DHSS in the shape of the
NHS for the future, and that all the distortions listed above will
continue, at least until such time as the financial situation changes.
It appears that the health and welfare services are expected to undergo
a period of retrenchment until such time as more money may be
available for their development. This money might become available
from (1) a greater proportion of the gross national product devoted to
the NHS, or (2) from the surplus wealth created by the next financial
boom. But there are severe limitations in either possibility. If a greater
proportion of the GNP were really to be allocated to the NHS, then this
might in fact detract from other areas of public spending that
contribute more positively to the health of the population, e.g.,
housing, education, employment. In addition, there are serious health
implications attendant on fast economic growth in itself, and growing
evidence that the increasing levels of stress, pollution and general
life-style necessary for such growth cause tremendous excess mortality
and morbidity in themselves.

Furthermore, if and when more money actually is available to the
services, the present decision-making and power structures will ensure
that the money is distributed in exactly the same manner as previously.
This will exacerbate the distortions in the NHS and fail to correct any
of the adverse effects on the people for whom the services are intended.

*Thus, whatever the financial situation of the country as a whole, or
the health services in particular, a change of shape in the NHS is
essential. Furthermore, this study shows that such a change of shape
is impossible without a change in the relationships of power within the
NHS, such that the interests of the community as a whole are
adequately represented.*

Recommendations

The problem remains how to change these power relationships in
practice. It would be too easy to be like the bystander who, asked how
he would get to a certain village, replied, 'Well, I wouldn't start from
here.' We must start from 'here', with the structure and the dynamics
of the health service as they are and certainly in need of radical change.
Any change that does occur will necessarily involve a period of
uncertainty and will need a very clear vision of the purpose of change
and a commitment to the ideals for the future.

Those who point out (rightly) that the shape and dynamics of the health service are simply mirrors of the shape and dynamics extant in society must be challenged when they therefore regard attempts at change in the NHS as useless until such time as the rest of society changes in shape. But the analysis of, and a change within, the health services can serve both to illuminate, and to catalyse real changes in, the rest of society.

To this end, consider the following positive proposals:

(1) The current period of economic stringency should be used positively to examine not only the effectiveness of particular medical interventions and practices, but also the effectiveness of the whole of the NHS in its present shape and the effect of the present relationships of power within the NHS.

(2) The entire NHS should be enabled to move in a direction that would increase its responsiveness to the needs of individuals and communities. The basic tenets of the services of the future should be that individuals must be encouraged to gain increasing control over their own bodies and that communities of 'consumers' should be able to take decisions regarding the services that are supposed to serve them.

(3) Government should have an enabling role not a management or service delivery function. It is clear that the greater proportion of the funds available to the services are in fact tied up from one year to the next in inescapable commitments to the functioning of the NHS in its present form. However, even the comparatively small percentage that is available for flexible use represents a large amount of money, and this must be used for real innovation. This should include innovations in the development of services which do not correspond to the current practice, but which explore some new shapes of service and which are dependent on different relationships of power within the NHS.

INDEX

113